HOW TO COOK STEAK

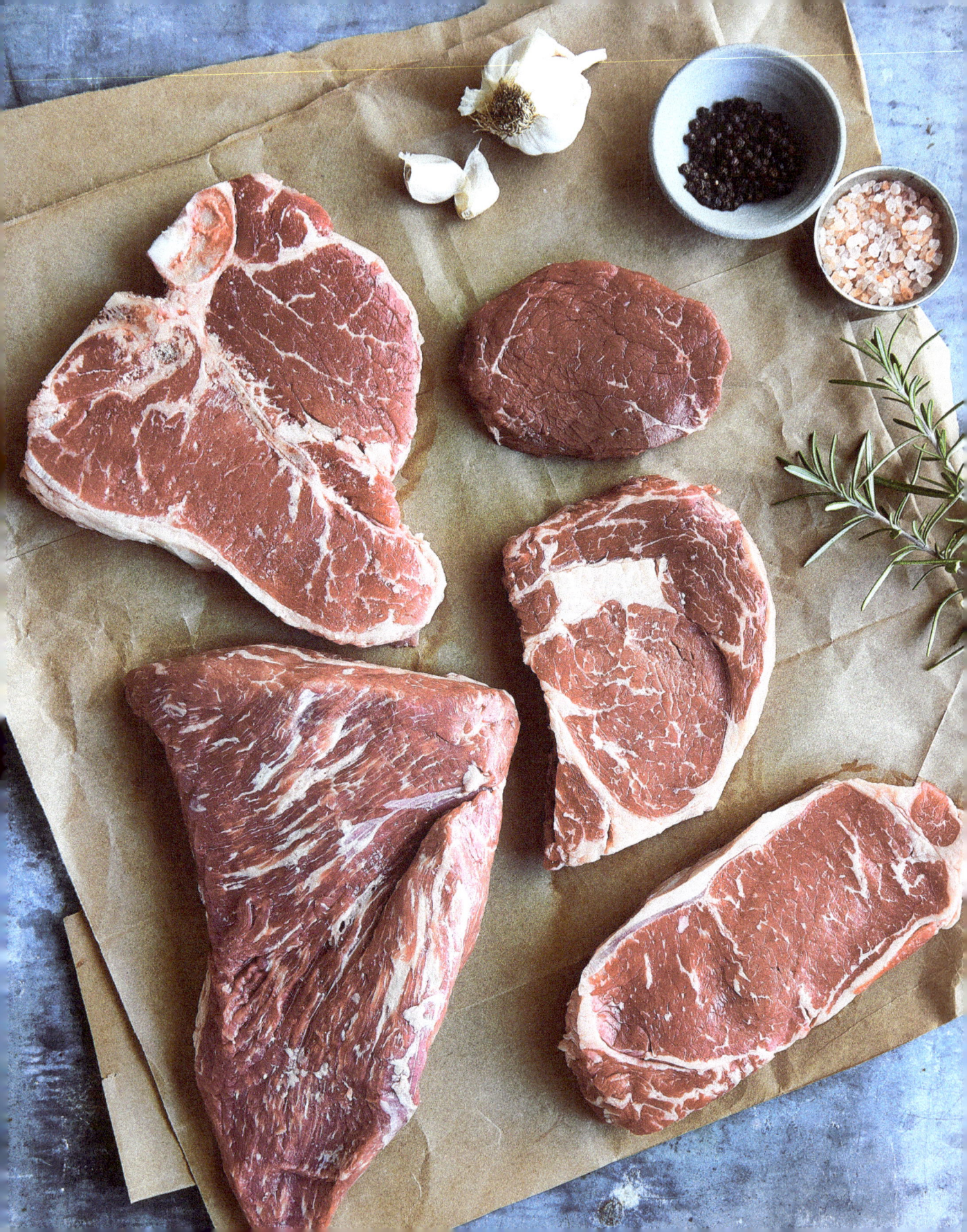

HOW TO COOK STEAK

Techniques to Master Selecting, Preparing, and Cooking Steak

Amanda Mason

Photography by Hélène Dujardin

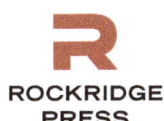

ROCKRIDGE PRESS

Copyright © 2021 by Rockridge Press, Emeryville, California

No part of this publication may be reproduced, stored in a retrieval system, or transmitted in any form or by any means, electronic, mechanical, photocopying, recording, scanning, or otherwise, except as permitted under Sections 107 or 108 of the 1976 United States Copyright Act, without the prior written permission of the Publisher. Requests to the Publisher for permission should be addressed to the Permissions Department, Rockridge Press, 6005 Shellmound Street, Suite 175, Emeryville, CA 94608.

Limit of Liability/Disclaimer of Warranty: The Publisher and the author make no representations or warranties with respect to the accuracy or completeness of the contents of this work and specifically disclaim all warranties, including without limitation warranties of fitness for a particular purpose. No warranty may be created or extended by sales or promotional materials. The advice and strategies contained herein may not be suitable for every situation. This work is sold with the understanding that the Publisher is not engaged in rendering medical, legal, or other professional advice or services. If professional assistance is required, the services of a competent professional person should be sought. Neither the Publisher nor the author shall be liable for damages arising herefrom. The fact that an individual, organization, or website is referred to in this work as a citation and/or potential source of further information does not mean that the author or the Publisher endorses the information the individual, organization, or website may provide or recommendations they/it may make. Further, readers should be aware that websites listed in this work may have changed or disappeared between when this work was written and when it is read.

For general information on our other products and services or to obtain technical support, please contact our Customer Care Department within the United States at (866) 744-2665, or outside the United States at (510) 253-0500.

Rockridge Press publishes its books in a variety of electronic and print formats. Some content that appears in print may not be available in electronic books, and vice versa.

TRADEMARKS: Rockridge Press and the Rockridge Press logo are trademarks or registered trademarks of Callisto Media Inc. and/or its affiliates, in the United States and other countries, and may not be used without written permission. All other trademarks are the property of their respective owners. Rockridge Press is not associated with any product or vendor mentioned in this book.

Interior and Cover Designer: Regina Stadnik
Art Producer: Samantha Ulban
Editor: Anna Pulley
Production Manager: Michael Kay
Production Editor: Melissa Edeburn

Photography © 2021 Hélène Dujardin. Food styling Anna Hampton. Illustrations © 2021 Tom Bingham. Author Photo courtesy of Brad Reed Photography.

ISBN: Print 978-1-64876-113-3
eBook 978-1-64876-114-0
R0

To Holly, Jennifer, Lyndsay, Tyree, Anthony, and Tyler—thank you for always being there, always supporting me, and continually encouraging me to dream bigger.

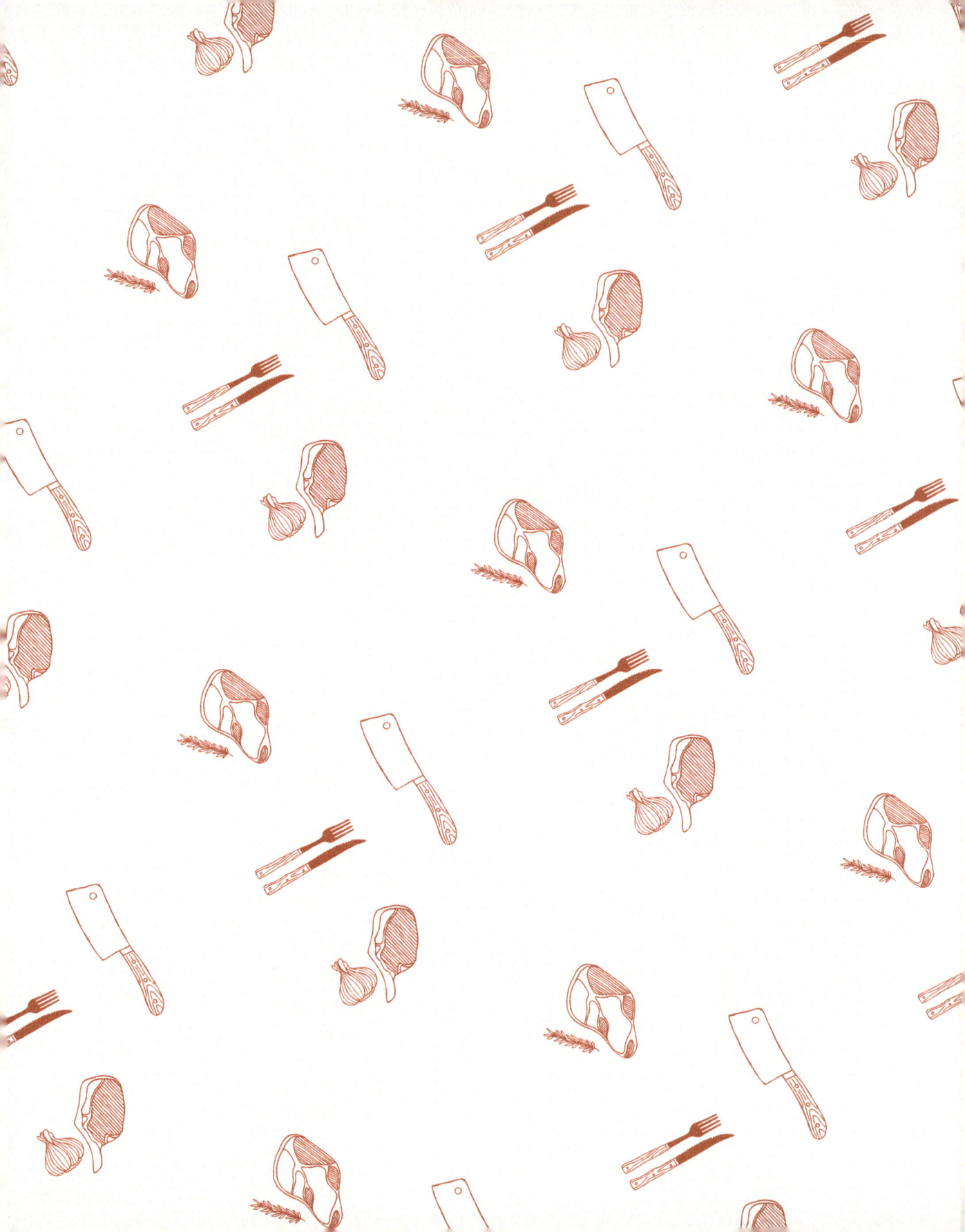

Contents

Introduction ix

PART ONE:
GETTING STARTED 1
   1: STEAK KNOW-HOW 3

PART TWO:
MAKING STEAK AT HOME + RECIPES 13
   2: SHOP, PREP, AND STORAGE 15
   3: ON THE GRILL AND STOVETOP 27
   4: OTHER COOKING METHODS 39

PART THREE:
MORE RECIPES 47
   5: PREMIUM STEAKS 49
   6: BUTCHER STEAKS 73
   7: OTHER STEAKS 97
   8: SIDES AND SAUCES 111

Measurement Conversions **129**

Index **130**

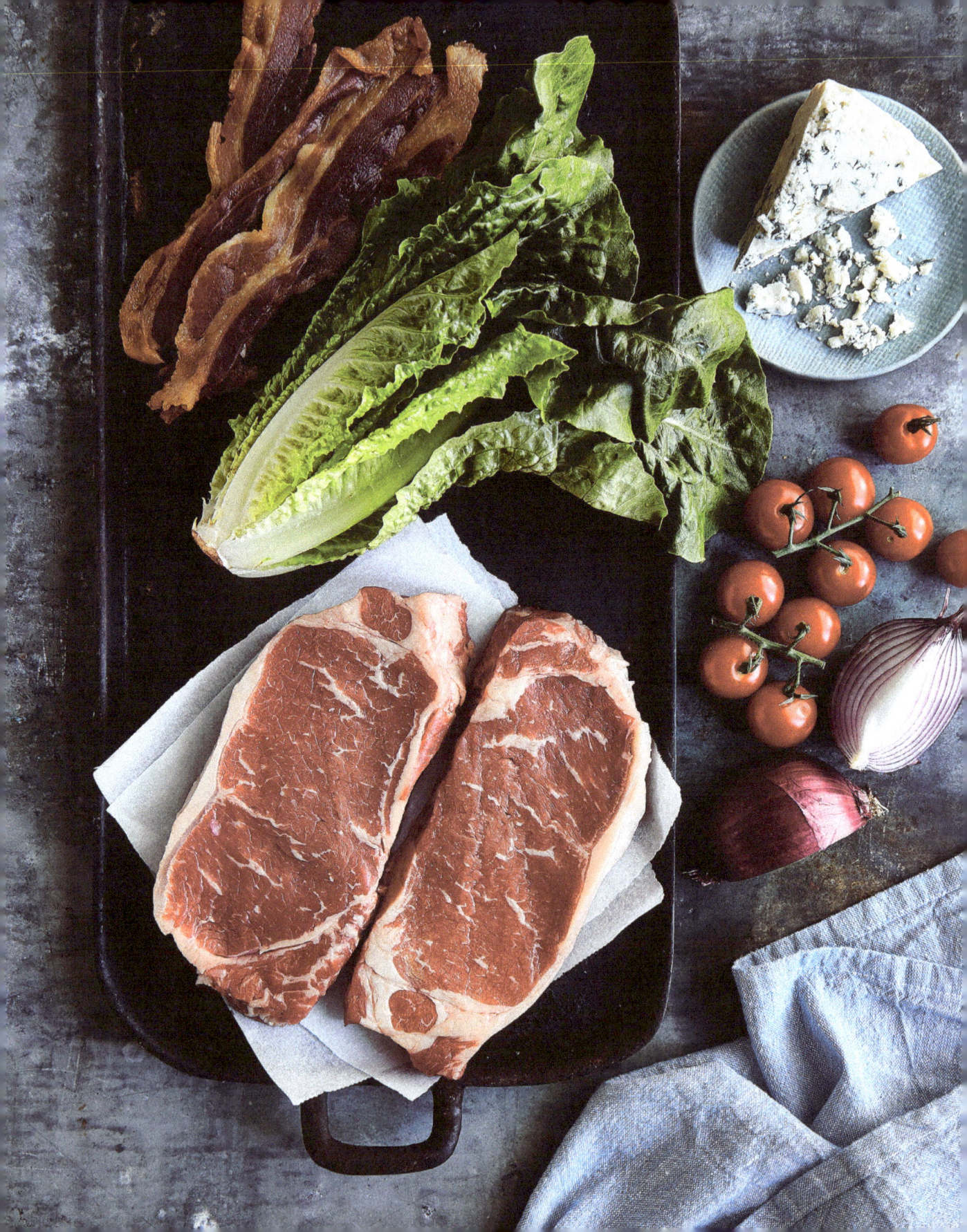

Introduction

I really wish there had been a book like this when I was learning to cook steak. I'm a Southern girl who grew up in Tennessee. My mom and grandmother had me in the kitchen cooking at an early age. By the time I was eight years old, I was making homemade buttermilk biscuits and scrambled eggs. But cooking steak was a completely different story. I didn't even attempt it until my early 20s—the first time was when I wanted to surprise my boyfriend with a grilled steak dinner. While he was at work, I prepared the ingredients and lit his grill. And I was scared! What if I undercooked the steak and we got sick? What if it was dry and tasted horrible? What if his house caught fire because I didn't really know how to use a grill? Despite these fears, the steak turned out tasty, and he was impressed with the results.

It's been more than 20 years since I made that first steak, and I'm here to tell you that cooking steak is easy. I've mastered the different ways to cook steak, and now I'm excited to teach you.

In part 1, we'll go over all the steak basics. Part 2 focuses on steak cooking methods. In part 3, you'll find recipes to apply your new knowledge to create delicious meals that will impress friends and family—and yourself.

Cooking steak is a skill that will serve you well for a lifetime. So, let's dive in!

PART ONE

GETTING STARTED

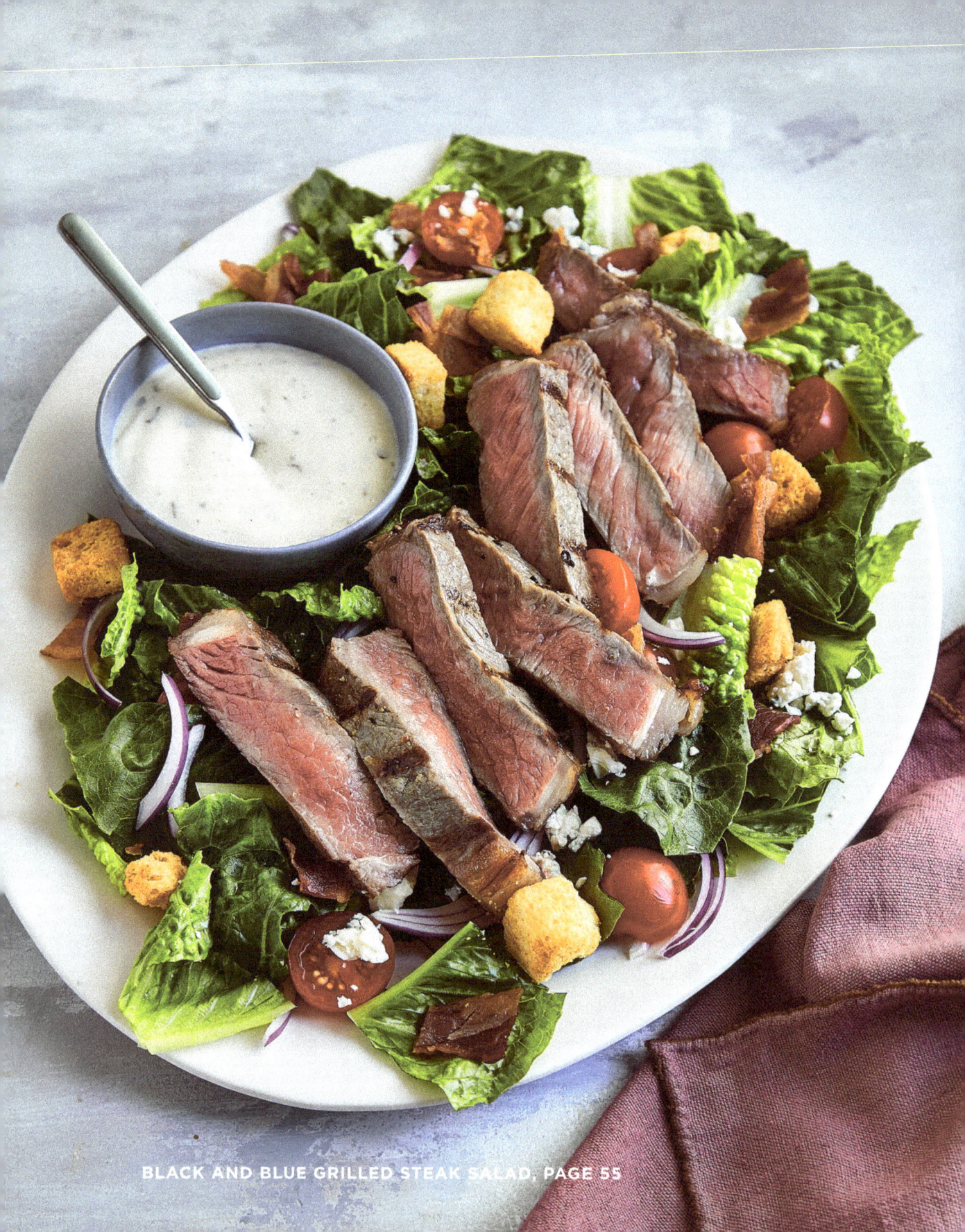
BLACK AND BLUE GRILLED STEAK SALAD, PAGE 55

CHAPTER 1
STEAK KNOW-HOW

In the following pages, we'll go over the different cuts of steak, the defining characteristics of each, and price points. You'll also learn where each cut comes from on the animal, which will help you determine cooking method and heat as well as cook time.

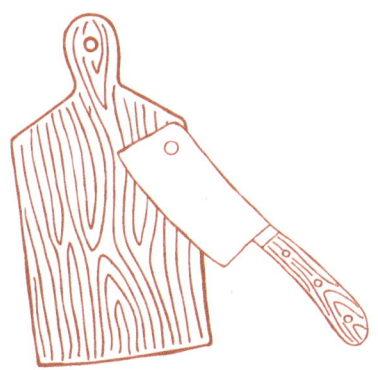

What Is Steak?

Let's define the word *steak*. It might seem odd to define something so obvious, but I'm doing it to prove a point. According to Merriam-Webster, a steak is "a slice of meat cut from a fleshy part of a beef carcass." But *steak* can also be used to describe non-beef meat (ham steak), a cross-section slice of a large fish (swordfish or tuna steak), ground beef (Salisbury steak), and even "a nonmeat food formed into a patty and cooked" (such as tofu, portobello mushrooms, or lentils).

In this cookbook, I've created 65 steak recipes that mostly follow the first definition, and what many of us think of when we think of steak, including filet mignon, porterhouse, rib eye, and T-bone. But I also include a few less common varieties, such as Salisbury steak, chicken-fried steak, pork steak, even a couple of vegan options.

Steak Cut Profiles

Understanding where meat comes from on the animal can help you make informed decisions about how to cook your steaks, at what degree of heat, and for how long. Premium cuts come from the top half of the animal and are considered higher quality, mainly because they're heavily marbled (that is, they have fat) and are tender. The premium cuts are filet mignon, New York strip, porterhouse, rib eye, T-bone, and tenderloin. These cuts tend to be relatively expensive mostly because of consumer demand, but age and tenderness are also factors.

Butcher's steaks are cuts that include flank, hanger, flat iron, sirloin, skirt, and tri-tip. These steaks come from the lower half of the cow. Although less expensive, they are still quite popular and tasty.

Let's look at the defining characteristics, prices, and best cooking methods for these cuts.

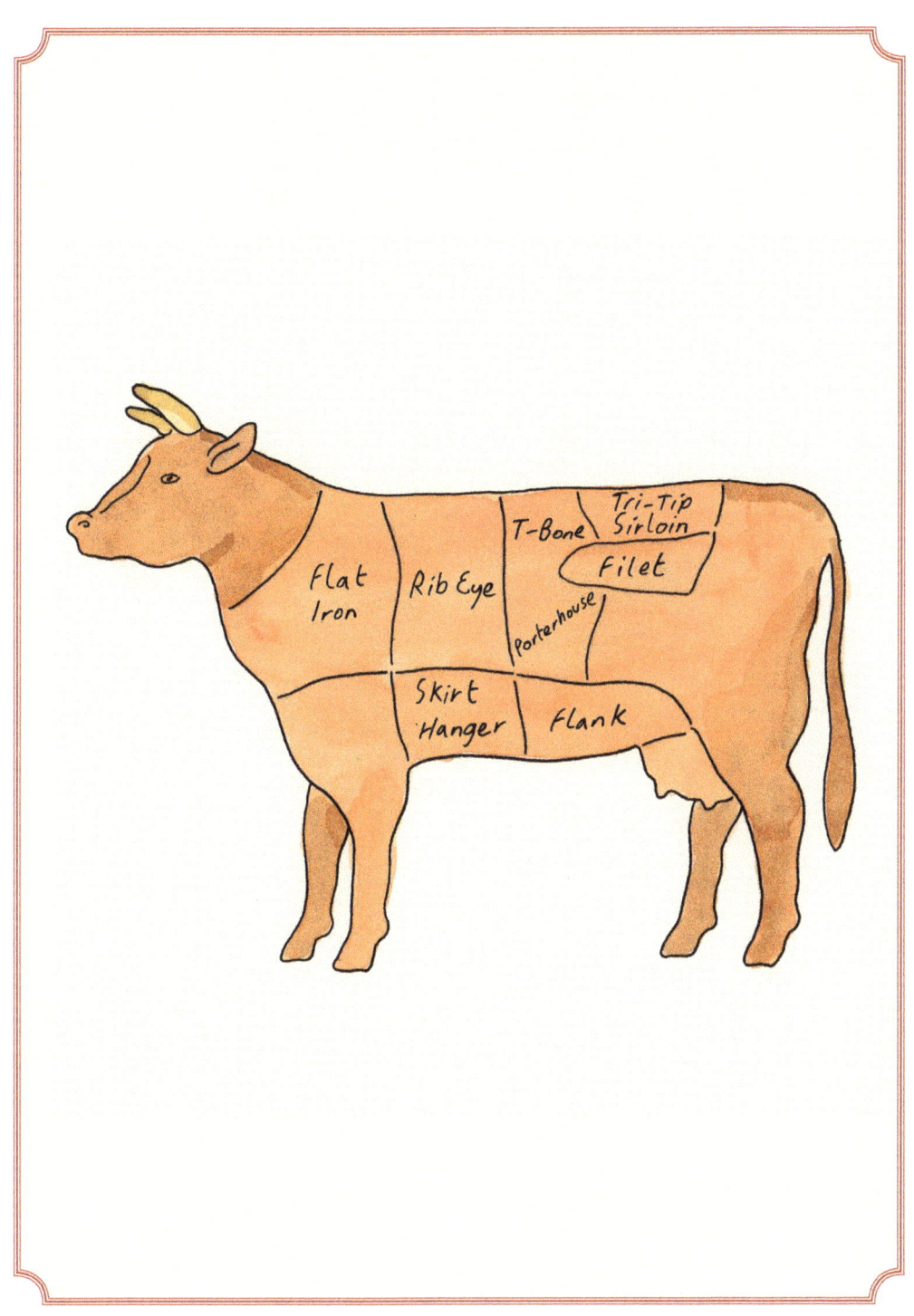

RIB EYE

COMES FROM: The rib portion

AKA: Cowboy cut, cowboy rib eye, deckle steak, Scotch fillet

DEFINING CHARACTERISTICS: This thick, juicy cut of meat, which is tender and heavily marbled, comes from ribs 6 through 12. When sliced, the rib bone is still attached.

BEST COOKING METHODS: Grill, pan-sear, stovetop-to-oven method, sous vide

PRICE: $$$

RECIPES: Creamy Steak Alfredo Pasta (page 61), Deep-Fried Boneless Rib Eye (page 43), Philly Cheesesteak Sandwiches (page 56), Mongolian Beef (page 58), Montreal Grilled Rib Eye with Sautéed Balsamic Mushrooms and Onions (page 68), Sous Vide Rib Eye Steaks with Sautéed Mushrooms and Balsamic Vinegar Sauce (page 62), Southwestern Steak Stew (page 60).

A rib eye steak comprises three areas: the bone, a large "eye" of meat attached to the bone, and the rib eye cap. The cap is the *spinalis dorsi* muscle, and many consider it the tastiest part of this steak—thus it tends to be expensive. You'll find this cut either as a round, whole muscle that has been trimmed, or in long strips about 1 inch thick. The cap has the tenderness of a filet mignon but the juiciness and flavor of a rib eye. Caps are best cooked on extremely high heat.

FILET MIGNON

COMES FROM: The short loin, which is behind the kidney, comes from the hip bone to the 13th rib.

AKA: Beef tenderloin, Chateaubriand, tenderloin roast, tenderloin steaks, whole filet

DEFINING CHARACTERISTICS: Long, boneless, thick cut. When sliced, the filets should have a universal dark pink-reddish color and thin streaks of fat running throughout. Filet mignon is one of the thickest cuts of steak and is juicy and tender.

BEST COOKING METHODS: It's best to cook beef tenderloin and individual filets on either high or medium-high heat. Cook a tenderloin roast in the oven. Pan-sear, grill, or use the stovetop-to-oven method for individual steaks.

PRICE: $$$

RECIPES: Garlic-Rosemary Filet Mignon (page 30), Garlic-Herb Roasted Beef Tenderloin (page 66), Pan-Seared Filet Mignon (page 37), Slow Cooker Garlic-Herb Filet Mignon and Potatoes (page 69), Steak Diane (page 64), Steak Tartare (page 45)

T-BONE/PORTERHOUSE

COMES FROM: This cut comes from the short loin.

AKA: Date steak

DEFINING CHARACTERISTICS: T-bone and porterhouse steaks have a T-shaped bone with meat on each side. Porterhouse is cut from the bottom area of the loin. T-bone is cut from the top and contains a smaller cut of tenderloin (filet mignon) and a long cut (New York strip) on the other side. The porterhouse typically has a larger tenderloin cut than the T-bone. According to United States Department of Agriculture (USDA) regulations, the tenderloin must be 1¼ inches wide to be classified as a porterhouse or ½ inch wide to be classified as a T-bone.

BEST COOKING METHODS: Both cuts cook well with dry heat cooking methods, such as grilling or broiling. The bone conducts heat, which helps the meat cook evenly and not dry out while cooking.

PRICE: $$$

RECIPES: Porterhouse Steak with Creamy Peppercorn-Mushroom Sauce (page 52), T-Bone Steak with Béarnaise Sauce (page 51)

SIRLOIN

COMES FROM: This cut comes from just behind the short loin. Several types of steaks are cut from the sirloin area. Top sirloin is the most tender part, whereas bottom sirloin is a larger cut, but not as tender.

AKA: Beef sirloin steak, petite sirloin, rump, sirloin steak, sirloin tip roast, top sirloin

DEFINING CHARACTERISTICS: A boneless cut, sirloin is lean and high in protein. It contains a lower amount of fat and marbling than other cuts, yet it is tender, juicy, and flavorful.

BEST COOKING METHODS: Any. This cut tastes great when marinated and grilled or pan-seared over high heat. It's also excellent cooked sous vide or deep-fried.

PRICE: $$

RECIPES: Classic Beef Stroganoff (page 91), Ginger-Soy Sirloin Steak Roll-Ups (page 74), Lemon-Pepper Petite Sirloin (page 33)

TRI-TIP

COMES FROM: This cut comes from the tip of the bottom of the sirloin.

AKA: Bottom sirloin, culotte, California's cut, Newport steak, Santa Maria steak, sirloin butt, sirloin tip, top sirloin. Tri-tip used to be thought of as waste, as there is only one cut per side of beef. Butchers would sometimes use it as stew meat. It's now a popular cut in high demand.

DEFINING CHARACTERISTICS: Small and triangular, tri-tip is one of the more tender cuts and is full of flavor. Even though it is a leaner cut, it does contain some fat, which contributes to the juiciness and tenderness of the steak. You can buy a whole tri-tip roast or have it cut into steaks. This cut of meat readily takes on the flavors of the ingredients it's marinated and cooked with.

BEST COOKING METHODS: Broiled, grilled, pan-seared, smoked

PRICE: $$

RECIPES: Grilled Tri-Tip with Chimichurri Sauce (page 80), Smoked Tri-Tip (page 94)

FLAT IRON

COMES FROM: This cut comes from the shoulder area.

AKA: Blade roast, book steak, butler steak, chuck clod, lifter roast, lifter steak, oyster blade steak, petite steak, top blade filet, shoulder top blade roast, top blade steak, top boneless chuck, triangle roast

DEFINING CHARACTERISTICS: Rectangular and nicely marbled, with a rich, beefy flavor. Flat iron steak is extremely tender and juicy. It's a versatile piece of meat and tends to take on the flavors of the ingredients with which it's combined.

BEST COOKING METHODS: High heat. It has a short cooking time, so grilling and pan-searing are great methods. It's the most tender and juiciest when cooked medium-rare (130°F to 135°F).

PRICE: $

RECIPES: Flat Iron Steak Stir-Fry with Asparagus and Red Pepper (page 84)

FLANK

COMES FROM: This cut comes from the abdominal muscles and lower chest.

AKA: Bavette, flank steak fillet, jiffy steak, London broil

DEFINING CHARACTERISTICS: A lean cut that contains little fat but is very flavorful, flank is deep red in color and consists of long muscle fibers. It's about a foot long and typically 1 inch thick. Most people cook the entire flank, then thinly slice it against the grain. This cut does a fantastic job of taking on the flavors of the ingredients it's paired with, which makes it an excellent choice for tacos and stir-fry.

BEST COOKING METHODS: Because it's such a tough piece of meat, flank benefits from being cooked either hot and fast or long and slow. The afterburner method (see page 28) works well for this cut. If you want a fast cook, grill it. If you want a slow cook, braise or smoke it. The goal in cooking this cut is to break down the connective tissues. It's best not to cook this steak past medium-rare because it will be chewy.

PRICE: $

RECIPES: Marinated Flank Steak (page 83), Grilled Flank Steak with Corn-Avocado Salsa (page 76)

SKIRT

COMES FROM: This cut comes from the plate (the cow's diaphragm muscle).

AKA: Arrachera, Romanian steak, Romanian tenderloin, Philadelphia steak

DEFINING CHARACTERISTICS: Often confused with flank steak (abdomen area), skirt (diaphragm) is a thin, long cut with a lot of connective tissue and tough muscle fibers. There are two parts to this cut: the inside and the outside. Most grocery stores sell the inside cut of the skirt because it's easier to prepare than the outside cut. Even though it has a good amount of fat, skirt is tougher to chew than flank. When prepared correctly, skirt has a wonderful beefy flavor, even more so than flank. You'll find that skirt does well marinated, especially in citrus juice, which helps break down the fibers before cooking.

BEST COOKING METHODS: Grilled or seared hot and fast

PRICE: $

RECIPES: Pressure Cooker Skirt Steak Fajitas (page 95), Spicy Southwest Cocoa-Rubbed Skirt Steak (page 86), Steak and Broccoli with Ramen Noodles (page 81)

HANGER

COMES FROM: This cut comes from the plate. It hangs between the rib and the loin, where it helps support the diaphragm.

AKA: Hanging tender, hanging tenderloin, lombatello, onglet, solomillo de pulmón

DEFINING CHARACTERISTICS: Often confused with skirt and flat iron steaks, hanger looks a lot like flank steak. It's V-shaped and considered one of the more tender cuts, even with the long membrane you can't eat running down the muscle. It contains a nice amount of marbling and is more tender than skirt and flank. Hanger steak does well when marinated in a citrus or vinegar base, and it has a uniquely delicious flavor when cooked correctly.

BEST COOKING METHODS: Grilled or broiled hot and fast

PRICE: $

RECIPES: Sweet and Spicy Grilled Hanger Steak (page 92), Chile-Lime Hanger Steak Tacos (page 90)

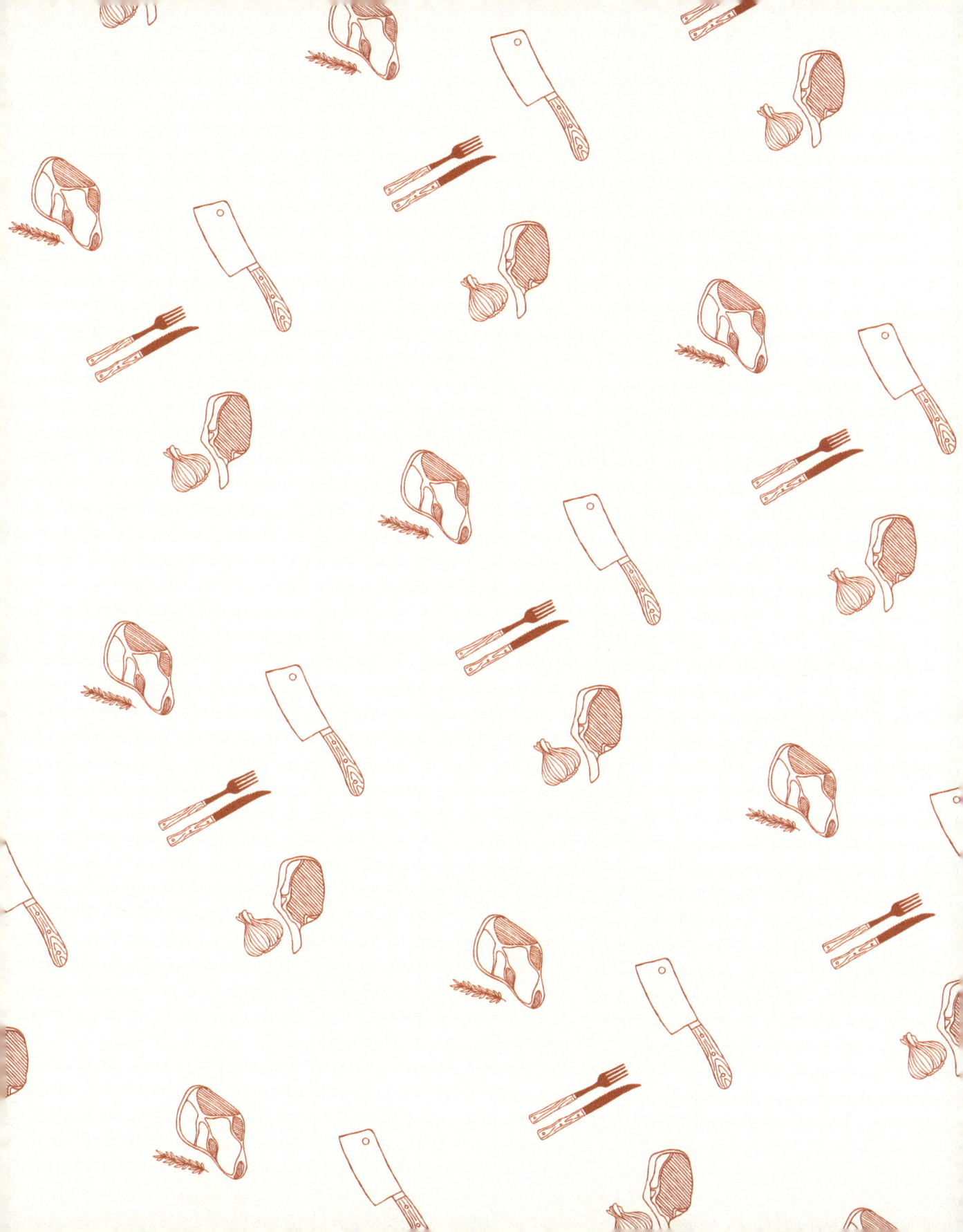

PART TWO

MAKING STEAK AT HOME + RECIPES

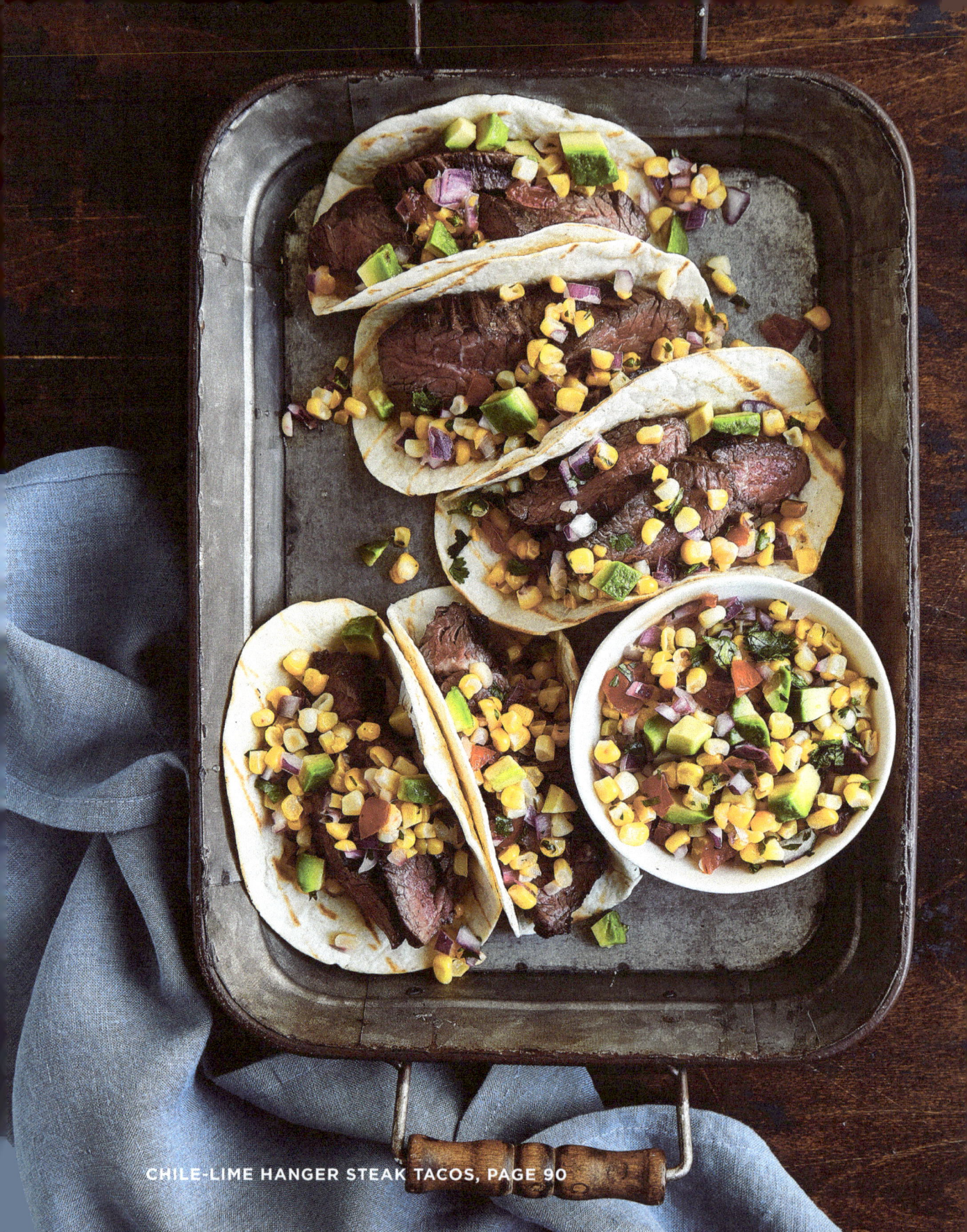

CHILE-LIME HANGER STEAK TACOS, PAGE 90

CHAPTER 2
SHOP, PREP, AND STORE

First, let's learn how to shop for steak. Understanding the different cuts and grades of meat will help guide your purchases. Then, we'll prepare the steak for cooking and talk about how to store it properly before and after it has been cooked. Once the steak is cooked, you may have leftovers, so it's important to know best practices for storing them. Finally, we'll take a look at ways to reheat steak so you can continue to enjoy every bite of juicy, tender goodness.

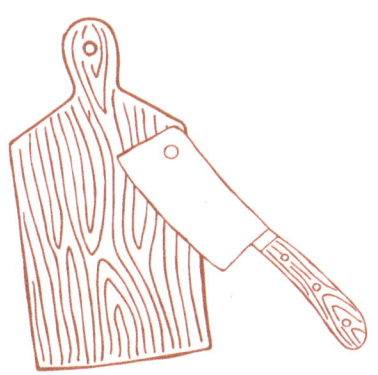

HOW TO TALK TO YOUR BUTCHER

When shopping at your local butcher shop or grocery store meat counter, you may encounter these terms:

BLACK ANGUS/CERTIFIED BLACK ANGUS: A popular meat thanks to its high degree of marbling, certified Angus beef comes from cattle that must have specific genetic qualities. According to the American Angus Association, Black Angus beef must also meet 10 strict criteria regarding muscling, fat, and size.

DRY AGING: A 30- to 40-day process that tenderizes meat by breaking down fat and removing moisture in a temperature- and humidity-controlled environment.

GRAIN-FED BEEF: Cows fed a diet of mostly corn and soy. A farmer can usually add weight to the cow more quickly when the cow is grain-fed.

GRASS-FED BEEF: Cows fed a diet of mostly grass. The cow tends to be smaller, and the meat contains less total fat than meat from a grain-fed cow.

KOBE: Beef from a particular strain of Japanese Wagyu cattle. This very expensive meat is prized for its tenderness and flavor.

NATURAL BEEF: Any meat that contains no artificial additives, flavorings, or preservatives.

ORGANIC BEEF: Cows that are fed a 100-percent organic diet, have not undergone genetic engineering, have free range to roam and eat, and have not been given antibiotics or hormones.

WAGYU: A luxury beef that comes from one of four specific breeds of Japanese cattle. It's heavily marbled, to the point that the meat is almost white and practically melts in your mouth.

How to Shop for Steak

Choosing a quality steak can be confusing and a little intimidating. There are a lot of choices to consider. Which meat grade? Grass-fed or grain-fed cows? Certified Angus beef, dry-aged beef, or Wagyu beef?

BEEF GRADES

The USDA designates eight beef quality grades, but for simplicity, we'll cover the three most common: **PRIME**, **CHOICE**, and **SELECT**. The grades are based on two main criteria: degree of marbling throughout the beef and estimated age of the cow at the time of slaughter.

USDA PRIME is considered the highest quality and yields tender, juicy, flavorful steaks from young, well-fed cows. Prime is also the most expensive grade. Only 2.9 percent of graded beef is considered Prime.

USDA CHOICE is the second highest quality and has a little less marbling than Prime. Choice is not as tender or juicy because of the reduced marbling. It's the most widely available grade in grocery stores; its price point is midway between Prime and Select.

USDA SELECT is the most frequently produced grade and contains relatively little fat. Select tends to be less flavorful because of the lack of marbling, and it's not as juicy or tender. It's also the least expensive option.

SENSORY CUES

Beef isn't required to have a grade, especially if it comes from a smaller butcher or local farm. Certain sensory cues can help you select a good steak.

A steak with a purplish hue indicates that the cow was recently butchered and the meat is extremely fresh. As the meat is exposed to oxygen, it turns that bright-red color we're used to seeing. You'll also likely see steaks that look brownish. According to the USDA, it's normal for fresh meat to change color during refrigeration, so there's no need to worry. Another visual indicator is marbling, which indicates that the steak will be tender and juicy.

Another important sensory cue is smell. A raw steak shouldn't have a strong, overpowering smell. If your steak has a pungent odor, it has spoiled and should be discarded.

OTHER KINDS OF STEAKS

As noted in chapter 1, the word *steak* can refer to fish, ham, ground beef, lamb, and tofu. This book includes recipes for Salisbury steak, grilled ham steak, tuna steak, lamb, and more. When making Salisbury steak, use any grade of ground beef you like; I recommend ground chuck because it's flavorful and readily available.

Building Your Steak Kitchen

To ensure your cooking experience is successful, let's look at some tools you'll need for the recipes in this cookbook, as well as basic pantry items you'll want to stock.

ESSENTIAL KITCHEN TOOLS

When setting up your kitchen, it's important to have the right tools to get the job done in the most efficient way. The good news is you may already have many of these tools on hand.

ALUMINUM FOIL: Use this foil to line baking sheets.

BAKING SHEETS: Use these sheets to let steaks rest before and after cooking and to cook side dishes.

BASTING BRUSHES: Use these tools to apply marinades and evenly distribute rubs on meat.

CAST-IRON SKILLET (13-INCH): Use this skillet for pan-searing and stovetop-to-oven cooking. Cast iron can handle high temperatures and does a phenomenal job maintaining heat.

CHEF'S KNIFE: A good chef's knife can be used for many tasks. It's great for mincing, slicing, and chopping vegetables. It can also be used when slicing meat and removing fat from steak.

CUTTING BOARDS: Use these boards for prepping meat and vegetables. I recommend having at least two cutting boards—one strictly for raw meat and the other for vegetables—to avoid cross-contamination.

DIGITAL MEAT THERMOMETER: Use this tool to gauge the internal temperature of meat while cooking.

OVEN MITTS: Use these mitts to reduce the risk of burning your hands and arms when reaching into the hot oven to remove meat, as well as when grabbing the handle of a hot skillet.

PARCHMENT PAPER: Use parchment paper when making compound butter and when lining baking sheets to make certain side dishes.

PARING KNIFE: Smaller than a chef's knife, the paring knife is great for peeling vegetables, slicing potatoes, and preparing garnishes.

PLASTIC BAGS (RESEALABLE, 1-GALLON SIZE): Use these bags for marinating meat and mixing ingredients, such as liquids or dry rubs.

TONGS: Use this tool for turning steaks and removing meat from dishes cooked on the stovetop or grill or in the oven. I keep at least two pair on hand.

NICE-TO-HAVE TOOLS

Although these tools are not necessary for cooking steak, they can allow you to try different types of recipes.

DEEP FRYER: This fryer can be used to cook certain cuts of steaks and make fries.

OUTDOOR GRILL: Use this tool to grill steaks outside.

PRESSURE COOKER: Quickly cook food with this sealed pot that uses steam to build pressure.

SMOKER: Use this piece of equipment outdoors to cook steak at a low temperature for a long period. (To convert a grill into a smoker, see the sidebar on page 29.)

SOUS VIDE PRECISION COOKER AND CONTAINER (12- OR 18-QUART): In the sous vide ("under vacuum") cooking method, you cook vacuum-sealed foods to a precise temperature in a water bath. The cooker attaches to the container and heats the water to the desired temperature.

VACUUM SEALER: This sealer is necessary for the sous vide cooking method. It also comes in handy when you want to marinate and freeze meat.

Pantry Must-Haves

Every home cook needs a well-stocked pantry. Keep the following ingredients on hand to make steak cooking easy anytime.

BROWN SUGAR (light and dark)

BUTTER (salted and unsalted)

GARLIC (fresh and powder)

OLIVE OIL

PEPPER (ground cayenne, coarse ground black, whole black peppercorns, red pepper flakes, ground white)

ROSEMARY (fresh and dried)

SALT (Himalayan, kosher, sea)

THYME (fresh and dried)

A Cut Above: Knife Skills to Know

When you hear the phrase "cutting steak" you may think about slicing into a steak you are about to devour, but it also applies to other purposes.

AGAINST THE GRAIN

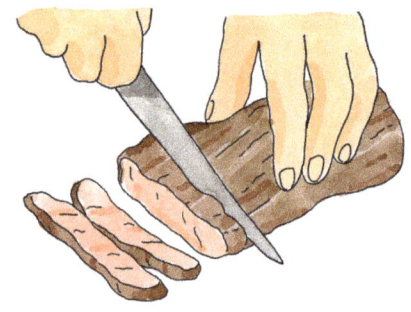

When slicing a cooked piece of meat, such as flank, hanger, or skirt steak, cut the meat against the grain. Muscle fibers are tough; cutting against the grain reduces the length of those fibers, making the meat easier to chew. To cut against the grain, first identify which direction the grain is running—look for parallel lines of muscle fibers running through the meat. Once you find the grain, cut perpendicular to it. I like to slice steak holding the knife at a slight angle to help break down those tough fibers. A chef's knife can be used when cutting steak against the grain.

TRIMMING FAT

When preparing individual steaks that contain a lot of extra fat (not marbling), trim away that fat to avoid unnecessary splatters during cooking. These splatters can result in burns and create a fire hazard. You can use a paring knife to trim fat, but a butcher's knife works best.

SEASONING AND MARINATING: THE BASICS

Seasoning

Always season steak both before and after cooking. But don't apply salt too far in advance. Salt extracts moisture and will start "cooking" the steak's exterior. How you cook the steak determines how you should season it, but simple is often best: I use coarse salt and black pepper.

Marinating

When it comes to marinating meat, aim for a minimum of 4 hours. I often recommend marinating between 12 and 24 hours. The longer the meat marinates, the more flavorful the result.

Brining

Two common ways to brine meat are wet brining and dry brining. The difference between the two methods is how the salt works. With a wet brine, meat is submerged in a salt-infused liquid. A dry brine works the opposite way and, when applied, draws moisture from the meat. A salt-based dry brine mixes with the remaining juices and is reabsorbed into the meat. There's no need to wet brine a quality steak because it's already tender and full of flavor. You're better off dry brining it because dry rubs penetrate the steak, producing additional flavor during cooking.

Scoring

Scoring steak helps when you have a tough cut, such as flank. It breaks down those long fibers that are hard to chew. Use a sharp knife to cut ¼-inch slits in the meat surface, then add seasonings and marinades.

Steak Doneness Chart

Some cooks test the doneness of a steak using their hands. My experience suggests the validity of this method. Here's how it works:

- Turn the palm up and relax one hand. Using the pointer finger of your other hand, touch the meaty pad right below your thumb. The pad should feel squishy. If you lightly touch a steak with your finger while it's cooking (you won't burn yourself if the touch is quick and light) and the steak feels squishy, its doneness is rare.

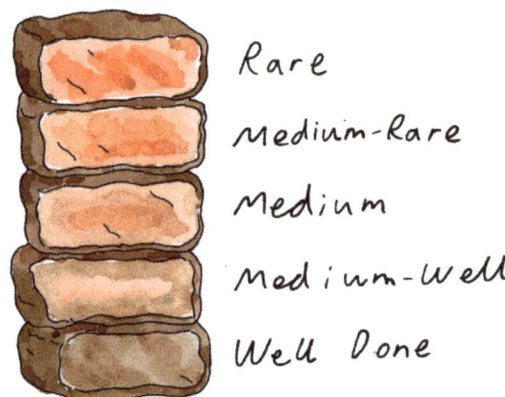

- Now, touch your palm right below your middle finger. If the steak feels like this area of your hand, its doneness is medium-rare.

- Now, touch right below your ring finger. If the steak feels like this area of your hand, its doneness is closer to medium.

- Lastly, touch the bottom of your palm right below your pinky. If the steak feels firm, like this area of your hand, its doneness is medium-well to well-done.

Although I feel comfortable using this method for a quick check, I don't recommend it when you're just learning to cook steak. Instead, use a digital meat thermometer to check the internal temperature to determine the level of doneness.

DONENESS	TEMPERATURE
Extra-Rare/Blue	80°F to 100°F (85°F to 105°F after resting)
Rare	120°F to 125°F (125°F to 130°F after resting)
Medium-Rare	130°F to 135°F (135°F to 140°F after resting)
Medium	140°F to 145°F (145°F to 150°F after resting)
Medium-Well	150°F to 155°F (155°F to 160°F after resting)
Well-Done	160°F+ (165°F+ after resting)

Wireless meat thermometers are great because you don't have to worry about the cord getting in the way. And although it's true that some juice escapes when the probe pierces the steak, that loss won't matter much if you're cooking a Prime or Choice cut (see page 17). I'd rather you get the doneness you desire.

For the most accurate internal temperature, insert the probe into the side of the steak and press it toward the center. The temperature will rise while the meat rests, so remove the steak from the heat when it registers 3 to 5 degrees below your preferred doneness. When it comes to pan-searing (see page 34), I rely on sear time to determine doneness.

How to Store Steak

If you plan to cook your meat within a couple days of purchase, you can safely refrigerate it in its original wrapping. Place the packaged raw meat in a large bowl or baking dish and store it on the bottom shelf of the refrigerator. The bowl is there in case the juices from the package leak—the last thing you want is bacteria growing in your refrigerator and contaminating other food.

Vacuum sealing is another popular choice for storing meat because it removes air but preserves moisture, which helps keep the meat tasting fresh when cooked.

You can also freeze raw meat. When I buy bulk meat, I remove it from the original packaging and put 4 or 5 pieces in a 1-gallon freezer-safe resealable plastic bag, which I place in the freezer. According to USDA guidelines, uncooked steaks can be frozen for up to 1 year.

When it comes to thawing frozen meat, safety is key. Place the frozen meat in a dish on the bottom shelf of the refrigerator to slowly thaw for 2 or 3 days before you plan to cook it. If you're in a hurry, you can safely place the packaged frozen meat in a large bowl filled with cold water. Change the water every 30 minutes so the meat thaws without temperature fluctuation, which can promote bacteria growth.

If you have leftover cooked steak, let it cool and then transfer it to an airtight container and store it in the refrigerator for up to 3 days.

HOW TO REHEAT STEAK

Steaks can be large, and you'll often have leftovers. It's important to know how to properly reheat leftover steak so it doesn't taste like a leathery brick. One of my favorite methods for reheating steak is to slowly warm it in the oven, then finish it off with a hot sear on the stovetop. Simply place the leftover steak in a cast-iron skillet or on a baking sheet and warm it in a preheated 250°F oven. Insert a digital thermometer into the side of the steak and, once the internal temperature reaches 110°F (25 to 30 minutes, depending on thickness), sear the steak in a skillet over high heat with 1 tablespoon of olive oil for 1 to 2 minutes per side.

Reheating steak in the microwave typically dries out the steak. To avoid this outcome, place the steak in a deep microwave-safe dish and pour 2 to 3 tablespoons of beef broth over it to maintain the moisture level. Set the microwave to medium heat and cook the steak in 20-second intervals, turning the dish at each interval, until it is warm.

About the Techniques + Recipes

Grilling. Searing. Broiling. Smoking. These are just some of the techniques for cooking steak that you'll learn and practice in the chapters that follow.

Many recipes include tips. Advanced technique tips will help you elevate your game. Make-it-easier tips help you save time and effort. Mix-it-up tips suggest cuts of steak that work well with a particular recipe. Prep tips offer efficiency advice and ways to avoid "mis-steaks." (See what I did there?) Lastly, some recipes offer substitutions for ingredients that may be hard to find.

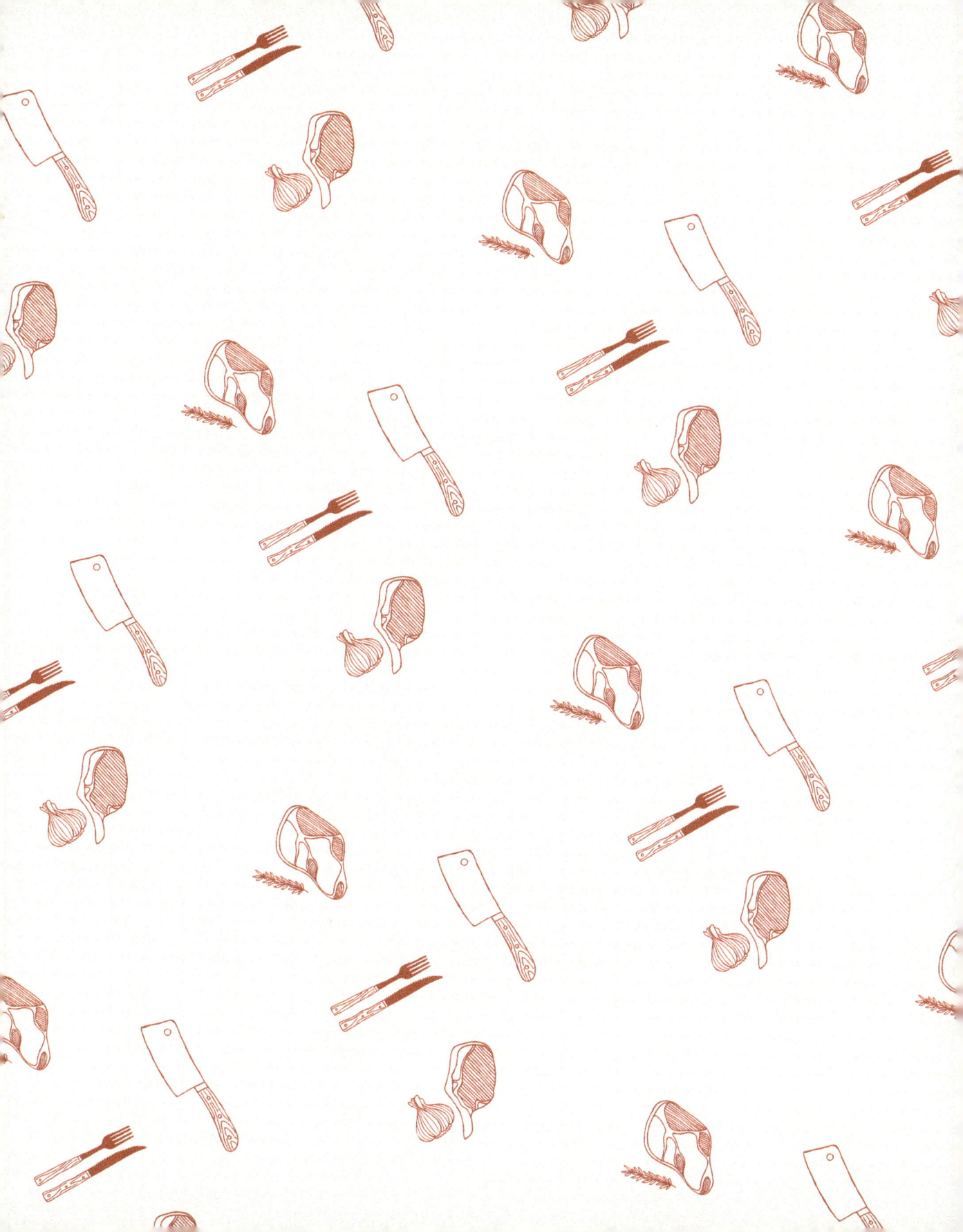

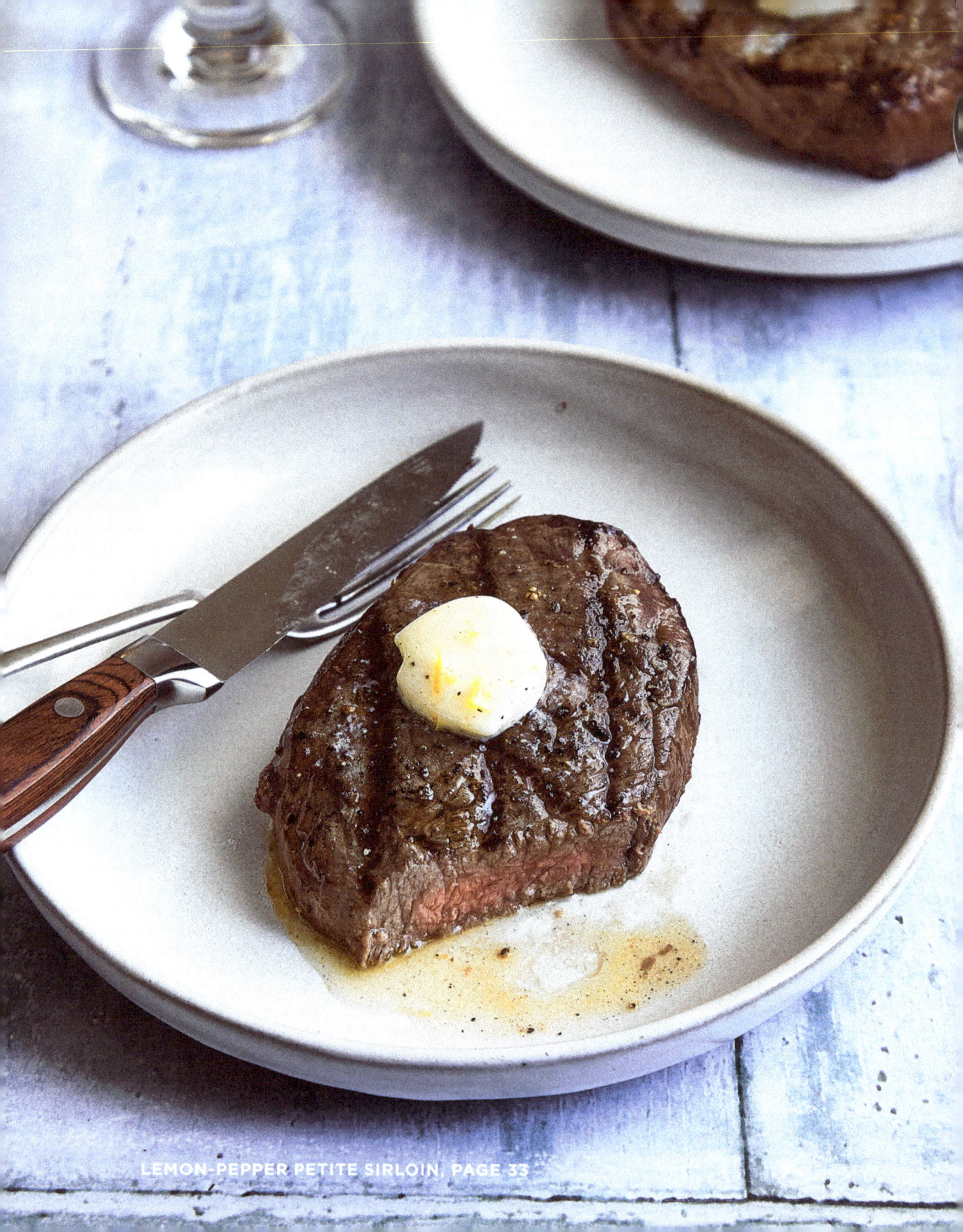

LEMON-PEPPER PETITE SIRLOIN, PAGE 33

CHAPTER 3
ON THE GRILL AND STOVETOP

30 Garlic-Rosemary Filet Mignon

33 Lemon-Pepper Petite Sirloin

37 Pan-Seared Filet Mignon

So, we've covered steak cuts, how to shop for steak, and how to set up your kitchen. Now let's discuss the best cooking methods. In this chapter, I cover grilling, pan-searing, reverse searing, sautéing, and broiling. I also include practice recipes so you can start cooking steak while you learn the techniques.

Outdoor Grilling

Grilling steak offers several benefits. First, you'll avoid ingesting the fat that renders from the meat and drips through the grates. Second, you can grill your sides and dessert (fruit!) with the meat. Third, you can avoid heating up your kitchen when you are trying to maintain a cool house during hot weather.

If using a **CHARCOAL GRILL**, heat the charcoals in a chimney starter. To do this, place the starter inside the grill directly on the grate. Crumple up 1 or 2 sheets of newspaper and put them in the chimney, then turn it upside-down. Fill the chimney three-quarters full with charcoal briquettes, then light the newspaper by applying a flame directly through the small slits at the bottom of the starter. When the briquettes are hot (orange and smoking), pour them onto one side of the grill so you can start a two-zone fire. Place the grill grate over the coals, close the lid, and let the grill heat to the desired temperature. When searing meat, place it on the grill grate directly over the coals. For indirect cooking, place the meat farther away from the coals.

If using a **GAS GRILL**, ensure the propane tank is securely in place, then open the grill lid, open the gas valve, and ignite the grill. Adjust the knobs based on your desired heat level, then close the lid. Let the grill heat to the desired temperature, then cook the meat on the grates.

When it comes to grilling steaks, there are a few methods. Here are the most common.

AFTERBURNER METHOD

This cooking method involves searing meat over an extremely hot flame the entire time the meat cooks. This method is great to use for single servings or when camping.

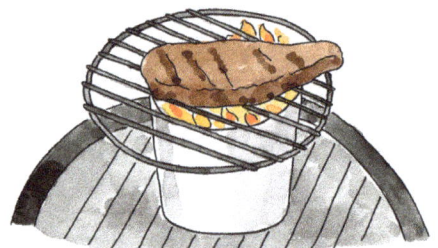

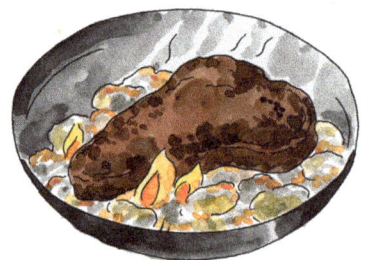

DIRECTLY OVER THE COALS

This method is exactly what it sounds like: placing meat directly on hot charcoals for a direct cook. This method imparts a delicious charbroil flavor, and it's also a way to cook meat quickly.

LOMO AL TRAPO, AKA GRILLED IN CLOTH

In this surprisingly easy cooking method, you wrap a salt-covered beef tenderloin in a wet cloth, secure it tightly with twine, then cook it directly on the hot coals until it reaches the desired doneness. The thick layer of salt forms a crust that coats the tenderloin so it can be cooked directly on the hot coals. Wrapping it in the cloth holds the salt in place, creating a flavorful crust.

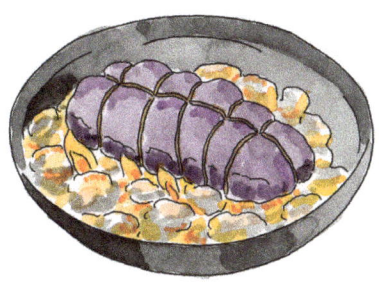

TURN YOUR GRILL INTO A SMOKER

If you don't own a smoker but want your steaks to have a smoky flavor, you can turn a standard charcoal grill into a smoker:

1. Remove the grill grate.
2. Heat charcoal briquettes in a chimney starter (about one-third full).
3. Once the coals are hot, place a disposable aluminum pan directly on one side of the wire rack inside the grill. Pour about 2 quarts of water into the pan.
4. Dump the hot charcoal briquettes onto the other side of the metal rack, stacking them.
5. Scatter a handful of wood chips (about 1 cup) on top of the briquettes.
6. Place the grill grate over the water pan and briquettes.
7. Insert a digital meat thermometer in the steak and place the steak on the grate directly over the water pan. Close the lid and open the vent about a quarter of the way to allow airflow.
8. Remove the meat once the thermometer reaches the desired temperature.

NOW YOU TRY

Let's start with an easy recipe using an outdoor grill. This recipe also works well using the lomo al trapo method (see page 29) if you opt to use a beef tenderloin instead of individual filet steaks.

GARLIC-ROSEMARY FILET MIGNON

In this preparation, filet mignon, one of the most delicious and tender cuts of meat, marinates in olive oil with fresh garlic and rosemary and is then grilled to perfection. This melt-in-your-mouth filet pairs beautifully with Homestyle Mashed Potatoes (page 114).

SERVES 4 / PREP TIME: 10 MINUTES, PLUS 4 HOURS 30 MINUTES TO MARINATE AND REST / COOK TIME: 15 MINUTES

10 garlic cloves, chopped

2 tablespoons chopped fresh rosemary leaves

4 (6-ounce) filet mignon steaks (about 1½ inches thick)

4 teaspoons sea salt

3 teaspoons coarse-ground black pepper

2 tablespoons olive oil

1. In a small bowl, stir together the garlic and rosemary.

2. Place the filets in a large glass dish. Generously season with the salt and pepper, firmly pressing the seasoning into both sides of the meat. Using a basting brush, apply the oil to both sides of each steak. Top the steaks with the garlic-rosemary mixture, lightly pressing it onto each steak. Cover the dish with plastic wrap and place in the refrigerator to marinate for at least 4 hours, or up to overnight.

3. Remove the plastic wrap and let the steaks rest at room temperature for 30 to 45 minutes.

4. Preheat a grill to high heat (about 400°F).

5. Place the steaks on the grill and sear for 2 to 3 minutes per side. It's okay if the garlic and rosemary fall off when you flip the steaks. Lower the grill temperature to medium-high (about 350°F). Insert a digital thermometer into the side of a steak and grill to your desired doneness. (See the chart on page 22 for temperatures.)

6. Transfer the steaks to a plate and loosely cover with aluminum foil. Let the steaks rest for 5 to 7 minutes before serving.

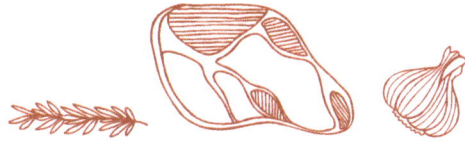

Stovetop Grilling

If you don't have an outdoor grill, you can use your stovetop to grill indoors. If you use the right kind of cookware, you can even achieve the coveted grill marks.

Start by placing a heavy grill pan or ridged cast-iron skillet over your stovetop burners, then set the heat to medium-high. Some grill pans cover two burners, which helps cook the meat more evenly. Allow the pan/skillet to preheat for 4 to 5 minutes. Then, using a basting brush, apply 2 to 3 tablespoons of oil or butter to the pan/skillet to help prevent the meat from sticking. Place the seasoned meat in the pan/skillet and cook for 2 to 3 minutes. Using tongs, flip the meat and allow it to cook until it reaches the desired level of doneness.

NOW YOU TRY
LEMON-PEPPER PETITE SIRLOIN

This flavorful steak is grilled on the stovetop, then topped with a delectable lemon-pepper compound butter.

SERVES 4 / PREP TIME: 10 MINUTES, PLUS 2 HOURS TO CHILL THE BUTTER / COOK TIME: 10 MINUTES

FOR THE LEMON-PEPPER COMPOUND BUTTER

- 8 tablespoons (1 stick) unsalted butter, at room temperature
- 1 tablespoon Himalayan salt
- 1 tablespoon coarse-ground black pepper
- 1 tablespoon grated lemon zest

FOR THE SIRLOIN

- 4 (4- to 6-ounce) petite sirloin steaks
- 4 teaspoons Himalayan salt
- 2 teaspoons coarse-ground black pepper

TO MAKE THE LEMON-PEPPER COMPOUND BUTTER

1. In a medium bowl, combine the butter, salt, pepper, and lemon zest. Using an electric mixer, mix on low speed until well combined. (Alternatively, you can use a handheld whisk.)

2. Transfer the butter to a small piece of parchment paper. Starting from one edge of the parchment, carefully roll the butter to form a log, then twist the ends of the parchment on both sides to seal. Refrigerate for at least 2 hours.

TO MAKE THE SIRLOIN

3. Season all sides of the steaks with the salt and pepper.

4. Heat a grill pan on the stovetop over medium-high heat. Add 1 tablespoon of compound butter to melt.

5. Working in batches, sear the steaks for 3 to 4 minutes per side for medium-rare, or to your desired doneness. Transfer the steaks to plates and top each with 1 tablespoon of compound butter to melt. Serve immediately. (Refrigerate the leftover compound butter in a resealable bag or an airtight container for up to 2 weeks.)

Stovetop and Oven Techniques

Cooking steak on the stovetop or in the oven is easy and convenient. And even though you can cook steak solely using one method or the other, together they offer the best of both worlds. By using the stovetop-to-oven technique, you can easily obtain a perfect crust on the outside with a tender and juicy texture inside. The best steaks for this cooking method are boneless cuts, such as rib eye. Simplified, the process involves searing a room-temperature steak in a very hot skillet, then broiling it in the oven until it reaches your desired doneness.

To use this method, preheat your oven's broiler. Then, heat an oven-safe skillet on the stovetop over high heat. Add olive oil or butter to the skillet and let it get very hot. Test it by tossing a pinch of water into the hot skillet—it should sizzle. While the skillet heats, pat the steak dry with paper towels. Generously season the steak on both sides with salt and pepper, then place it in the hot skillet. If cooking multiple steaks, make sure they are 3 to 4 inches apart. Sear the steaks for about 3 minutes per side. Transfer the skillet to the oven and broil for 3 minutes. Using tongs, flip the steak and broil for 3 more minutes for medium-rare, or to your desired doneness.

PAN-SEARING

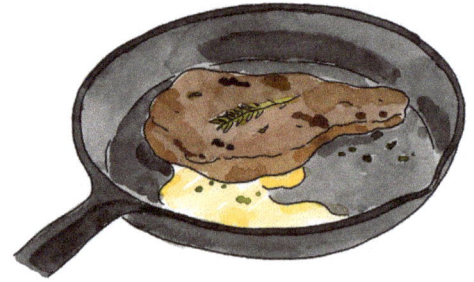

Pan-searing steak is all about building flavor. The technique is most often used to obtain a savory brown crust on the outside of steak. The process entails heating oil or butter in a skillet on the stovetop over very high heat, then adding the patted-dry and seasoned steak to cook for a few minutes on each side (3 to 4 minutes per side for medium-rare). Drying the steaks is important because if any moisture remains on the steak's exterior, it needs to evaporate before the meat can begin to brown. Generously seasoning the patted-dry steaks on both sides helps create a flavorful crust. The best candidates for searing are boneless quick-cooking steaks between 1 and 1½ inches thick, such as filet mignon, New York strip, or rib eye.

SAUTÉING

Often compared to pan-searing, sautéing is used to brown or cook food quickly over high heat using a small amount of oil or butter in a large pan. Sautéing differs from searing in that searing only browns the surface of the food, whereas sautéing cooks the food. Any cut of meat can be sautéed.

REVERSE SEARING

As its name implies, reverse searing is the opposite of the stovetop-to-oven method in that it involves slow-cooking a steak in the oven first, then finishing it off with a hot sear in a preheated skillet on the stovetop. If you're looking for a steak evenly cooked from edge to edge that still has a succulent crust, you'll want to use the reverse-searing technique. This technique works best for thick-cut Prime or Choice steaks, 1½ to 2 inches thick, as well as cuts with some marbling, such as filet mignon, New York strip, and rib eye. To apply this technique, season the steak, then place it in an oven-safe skillet in a preheated 250°F oven. Cook the steak until it's about 10°F below your desired doneness. While the steaks cook, heat a skillet over high heat until very hot. Transfer the steak to the hot skillet and sear for 1 minute per side for medium-rare, or to your desired doneness.

THE MAILLARD REACTION

Whether you know the term or not, you've eaten food that has benefited from the Maillard reaction, which occurs with all kinds of foods, not just meat. The Maillard reaction is a chemical reaction between amino acids and sugars that gives browned food its distinctive flavor. Not to be confused with caramelization, which is when only sugar is exposed to high temperatures, the Maillard reaction produces the dark brown, flavorful crust on a juicy steak. It starts at around 250°F and fully kicks in at around 300°F. It can be obtained only with the right temperature, acidity level, and moisture content. Getting meat as dry as possible before cooking is key.

BROILING

Your oven's broiler cooks food quickly by exposing it to high heat from a direct flame. Broiling does an excellent job of charring the edges of foods, achieving the perfect crust on a cheesy casserole, for instance, as well as making steak crispier. Fish, poultry, pork chops, vegetables, and some red meats are suitable for broiling. The temperatures used to broil are usually between 500°F and 550°F. Although often underutilized, broiling is a fast, simple process. Turn your oven to the broil setting and let it preheat for 5 to 10 minutes. Put the food on a broiling pan or in an oven-safe skillet, then place it directly under the broiler until it reaches your desired doneness. It helps to spread out the food while broiling so the surface is exposed to the heat for more even cooking and browning.

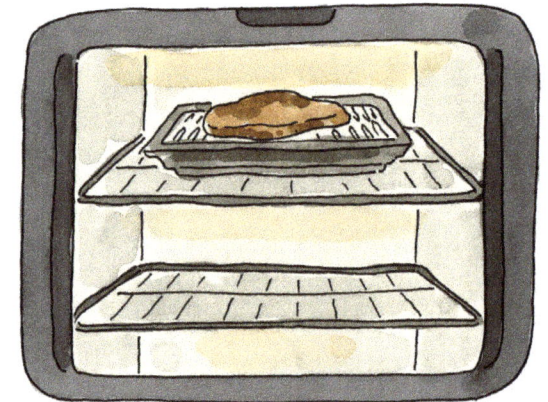

NOW YOU TRY
PAN-SEARED FILET MIGNON

The Maillard reaction (see page 35) is easy to achieve when you pan-sear filet mignon in olive oil. The fresh garlic, thyme, and rosemary add flavor and aroma, and when the butter caramelizes and you finish off the sear, you're left with a succulent steak, perfect for any occasion. For extra-special occasions, top the steak with my richly flavorful Smoky Hollandaise Sauce (page 124).

SERVES 4 / PREP TIME: 10 MINUTES / COOK TIME: 20 MINUTES

4 filet mignon steaks, at room temperature

4 teaspoons Himalayan salt

4 teaspoons coarse-ground black pepper

¼ cup olive oil

6 garlic cloves, peeled and lightly smashed

4 thyme sprigs

4 rosemary sprigs

2 tablespoons unsalted butter, cut into small pieces

1. Season the steaks with the salt and pepper, ensuring each side is evenly coated.

2. In a large skillet, heat the oil over medium-high heat for 3 to 4 minutes, until very hot.

3. Add the steaks and pan-sear for 4 minutes on one side to form the crust. About 2 minutes into the sear, scatter the garlic, thyme, rosemary, and half of the butter pieces in the skillet around the steaks. Flip the steaks and sear the other side for 5 to 6 minutes.

4. Add the remaining butter to the skillet. The butter should start to caramelize. Spoon the butter mixture over each steak several times.

5. Using tongs, slowly roll each filet on all sides to sear in the butter mixture. Transfer the steaks to a shallow dish. Let rest for 5 minutes before serving.

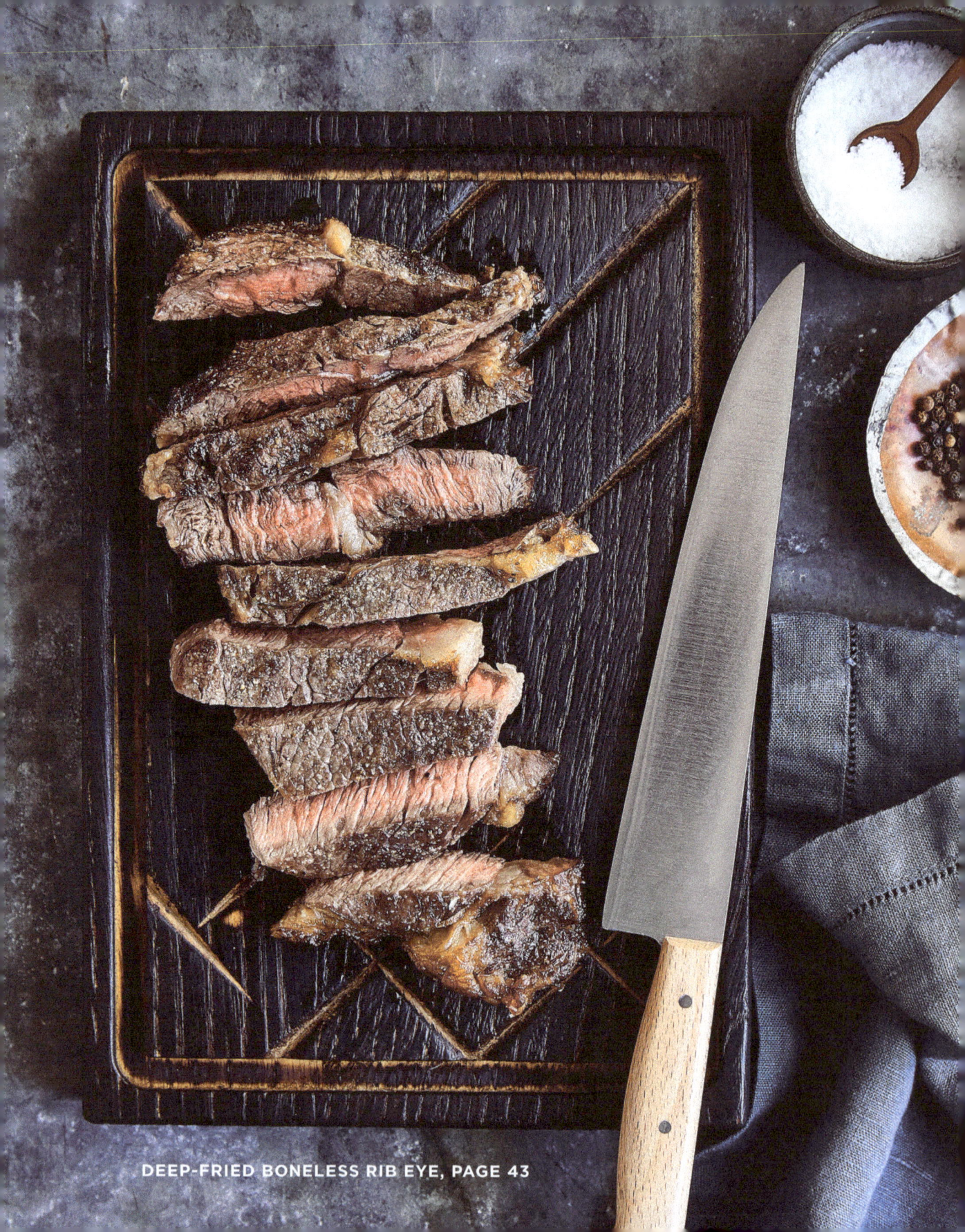

DEEP-FRIED BONELESS RIB EYE, PAGE 43

CHAPTER 4
OTHER COOKING METHODS

41   Sous Vide New York Strip Steak
43   Deep-Fried Boneless Rib Eye
45   Steak Tartare

Now it's time to look at a few less common, but no less effective, methods you can use to cook steak. In this chapter, we cover sous vide, deep frying, and even how to prepare steak tartare.

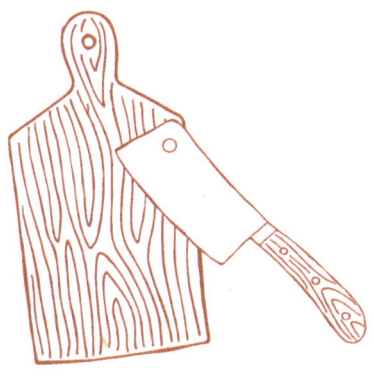

Sous Vide

One of my favorite ways to cook steak, sous vide is a cooking method that uses a temperature control to deliver the exact level of doneness every time. The sous vide method involves vacuum sealing foods, then cooking them in temperature-controlled water using a precision cooker device, which heats and circulates the water at a precise temperature. Sous vide used to be the domain of high-end restaurant chefs, but it has recently become popular for home cooks thanks to the availability and affordability of the required precision cooker. The method involves four easy steps, though you should reference your sous vide manual for specific instructions.

1. Use a vacuum sealer to remove the air and seal the meat, along with any seasonings you like, in a plastic bag.

2. Fill a large bin with water and securely attach the precision cooker to the bin. Set the time and temperature according to your desired doneness.

3. Place the sealed bag in the temperature-controlled water. Cook until the timer sounds to signal that the desired temperature is reached. Remove the meat from the bag.

4. In a hot skillet or grill, sear each side of the meat for 30 to 45 seconds to add a golden crust.

The beauty of sous vide is you can leave the meat in the temperature-controlled water for several hours and the internal temperature will remain the same and not overcook. You can use any cut of meat or thickness for sous vide, but the best results come with thicker cuts, such as filet mignon, New York strip, and rib eye. When grilling or pan-searing these cuts, it's harder to cook the center properly without overcooking the rest of the steak. The sous vide method delivers consistently cooked meats throughout.

Use the following chart time for the sous vide cooking method.

DONENESS	TEMPERATURE	TIME
Very Rare to Rare	120°F to 128°F	1 to 2½ hours
Medium-Rare	129°F to 134°F	1 to 4 hours (2½ hours for temperatures under 130°F)
Medium	135°F to 144°F	1 to 4 hours
Medium-Well	145°F to 155°F	1 to 3½ hours
Well-Done	156°F and up	1 to 3 hours

NOW YOU TRY
SOUS VIDE NEW YORK STRIP STEAK

This recipe is for one steak, regardless of its thickness. You will need a sous vide precision cooker, a 12- to 18-quart container, plastic cooking pouches, and a vacuum sealer.

SERVES 2 / PREP TIME: 15 MINUTES / COOK TIME: 1 HOUR

1 New York strip steak
2 teaspoons kosher salt, divided
1 teaspoon coarse-ground black pepper
1 rosemary sprig
2 garlic cloves, peeled and lightly smashed
1 tablespoon olive oil

1. Season both sides of the steak with 1 teaspoon of salt and the pepper.
2. Put the seasoned steak in a sous vide cooking pouch or vacuum sealer bag, then place the rosemary and garlic on top of the steak. Using a vacuum sealer, remove all the air from the bag and seal it. Set aside.
3. Fill the sous vide container with about 2 gallons of water. Securely attach the precision cooker to the container. Set the temperature to the desired doneness of the steak and set the timer.
4. Once the water reaches the desired temperature, place the vacuum-sealed bag in the water and cook until the timer sounds.
5. In a large skillet, heat the oil over high heat for 2 to 3 minutes, until very hot. Remove the steak from the bag and place it, along with the garlic and rosemary, in the skillet. Sprinkle the remaining 1 teaspoon of salt over the steak and sear for 1 to 2 minutes total, turning to ensure that the sides and edges are seared. Serve immediately.

Deep-Frying Steak

The saying is true: You can deep-fry just about anything—including steak! The most obvious example is chicken-fried steak. But if you haven't tried deep-fried rib eye or sirloin, you should. When seasoned properly, deep-frying steak produces an impressive and delicious crust. And if you like a medium-well to well-done steak, deep-frying is the way to go.

To deep-fry steak, you'll need a deep fryer or other heavy, deep pan and at least 2 quarts of an oil with a high smoke point, such as peanut or canola oil. Pour the oil into the deep fryer or pan; if using a deep fryer, the oil should come up to at least the minimum fill line. Heat the oil until it reaches 375°F. If using a deep pan, use a candy thermometer to check the oil temperature. Place the seasoned steak in the deep-fryer basket and lower it to completely submerge it in the oil, or put the steak directly into the oil in the pan. Once the prescribed cooking time has passed and the meat reaches your desired doneness, use tongs to remove it from the oil and place on paper towels to drain.

NOW YOU TRY
DEEP-FRIED BONELESS RIB EYE

Deep-frying steak forms a succulent crust and produces consistent results every time. It may seem like the seasoning is a bit heavy, but you need it to get that crispy, flavorful crust.

SERVES 2 / PREP TIME: 10 MINUTES / COOK TIME: 10 MINUTES

2 quarts peanut or canola oil

1 (6- to 8-ounce) boneless rib eye steak, at room temperature

1 teaspoon kosher salt

1 teaspoon coarse-ground black pepper

½ teaspoon garlic salt

½ teaspoon onion powder

1. Pour the oil into the deep fryer and heat until it reaches 375°F.
2. Season the steak on all sides with the salt, pepper, garlic salt, and onion powder.
3. For a 1-inch-thick steak, deep-fry for 4 to 5 minutes for medium-rare doneness. For a 1½-inch-thick steak, deep-fry for 8 to 10 minutes for medium to medium-well. (If you don't feel comfortable relying on time to determine doneness, insert a digital thermometer into the middle of the steak before placing it in the deep-fryer basket.)

> **PREP TIP:** The oil used for deep-frying can be reused, and there's no hard-and-fast rule as to how many times. The oil breaks down the more it's used, which is why I discard it after three uses. To store the oil for reuse, let it cool completely, then pour it through a mesh container into a large container, close tightly, and store at room temperature for up to 2 months.

Other Cooking Methods

Steak Tartare

Though technically not a cooking method, tartare is a versatile meat dish made from raw minced, ground, or finely hand-chopped beef and often served at high-end French restaurants. Also called "tiger meat," it's typically served raw but can also be lightly seared. Some people are concerned about the safety of tartare because it's raw. If in doubt, ask your butcher for assistance picking a fresh quality cut. A good-quality steak tartare is made with raw Prime meat served very cold and topped with a raw egg yolk. I enjoy serving steak tartare raw as an appetizer or even on a charcuterie board.

NOW YOU TRY
STEAK TARTARE

Although raw steak may not be everyone's cup of tea, steak tartare is considered a delicacy and is quite tasty. Plus, it's simple to make. I typically use ground filet mignon when making tartare. Ask your butcher to run the steak through a meat grinder. (Keep in mind that consuming raw or undercooked meat may increase the risk of foodborne illnesses and is not recommended for those who are immunocompromised.)

SERVES 2 / PREP TIME: 15 MINUTES, PLUS 30 MINUTES TO CHILL

- 8 ounces filet mignon, ground
- 5 garlic cloves, minced
- 2 teaspoons finely minced shallot, plus more if desired
- 2 teaspoons capers, whole or smashed, plus more if desired
- 2 teaspoons fresh tarragon leaves, finely chopped, plus more if desired
- 1 tablespoon Dijon mustard
- 1 teaspoon freshly squeezed lemon juice
- 1 teaspoon Himalayan salt
- 1 tablespoon coarse-ground black pepper
- 1 large egg yolk (optional)
- Crackers or Parmesan crisps, for serving

1. In a small bowl, stir together the filet, garlic, shallot, capers, tarragon, Dijon mustard, lemon juice, salt, and pepper.
2. Place a 2-inch round cookie cutter on a long dish. Pack the meat mixture into the cookie cutter. Gently remove the cookie cutter.
3. Place the egg yolk (if using) on top of the tartare.
4. Arrange additional capers, chopped tarragon, and minced shallot around the tartare, if desired. Refrigerate for 30 minutes to chill. Serve cold with crackers or Parmesan crisps.

> **PREP TIP:** Discard the egg white, or refrigerate it in an airtight container for up to 4 days for another use.

Other Cooking Methods

PART THREE

MORE RECIPES

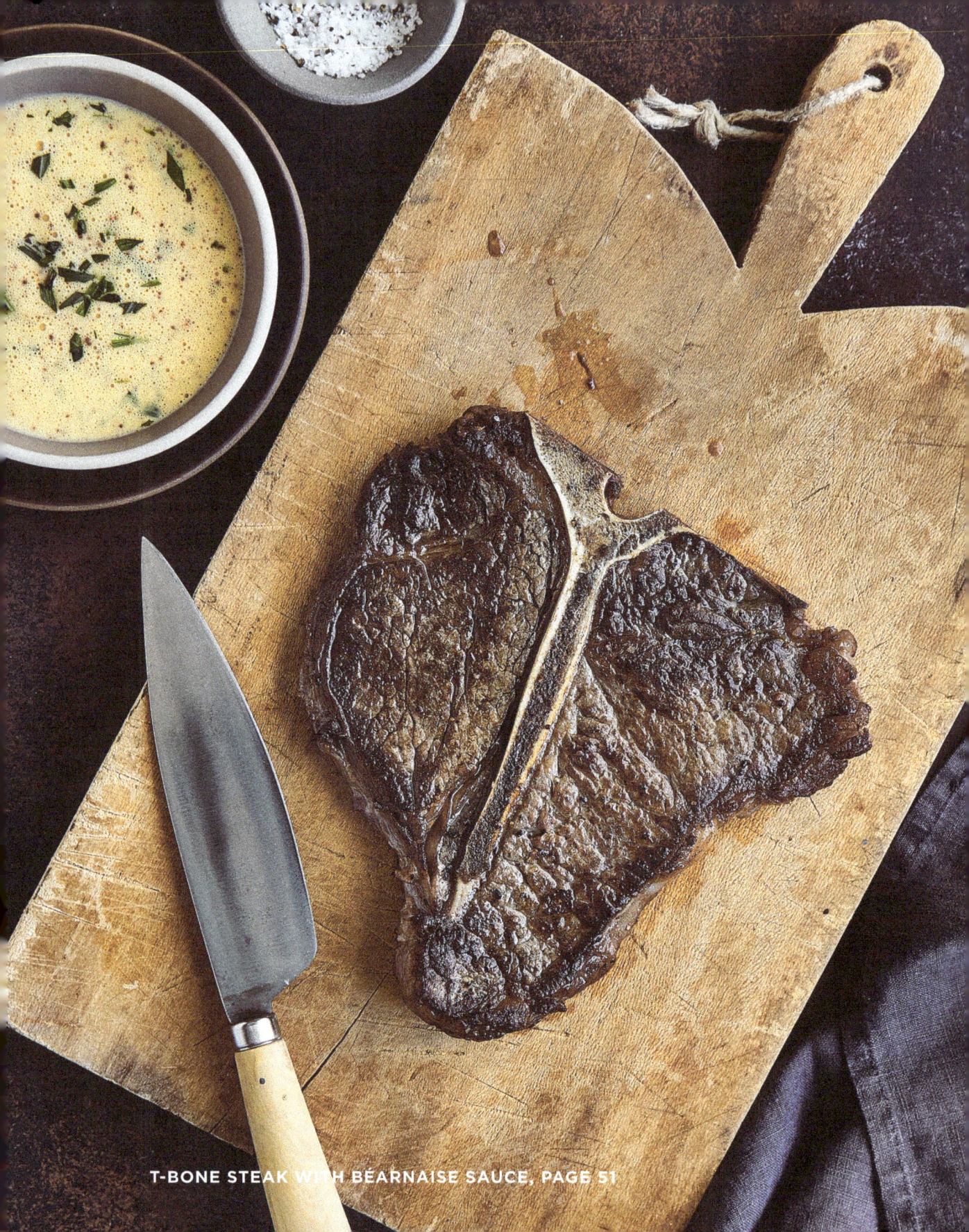

T-BONE STEAK WITH BÉARNAISE SAUCE, PAGE 51

CHAPTER 5
PREMIUM STEAKS

50 Pan-Seared New York Strip with Garlic-Rosemary Compound Butter

51 T-Bone Steak with Béarnaise Sauce

52 Porterhouse Steak with Creamy Peppercorn-Mushroom Sauce

54 Creamy Cajun Steak Bites

55 Black and Blue Grilled Steak Salad

56 Philly Cheesesteak Sandwiches

58 Mongolian Beef

60 Southwestern Steak Stew

61 Creamy Steak Alfredo Pasta

62 Sous Vide Rib Eye Steaks with Sautéed Mushrooms and Balsamic Vinegar Sauce

64 Steak Diane

65 Oven-Roasted Prime Rib with Horseradish Sauce

66 Garlic-Herb Roasted Beef Tenderloin

67 Slow Cooker French Dip Sandwiches au Jus

68 Montreal Grilled Rib Eye with Sautéed Balsamic Mushrooms and Onions

69 Slow Cooker Garlic-Herb Filet Mignon and Potatoes

70 Red Curry Steak and Vegetable Kebabs

PAN-SEARED NEW YORK STRIP WITH GARLIC-ROSEMARY COMPOUND BUTTER

This easy three-step method produces the perfect steak every time. We season the steak, pan-sear it to trigger the Maillard reaction (see page 35), then finish it in the oven. Using simple ingredients, this steak gets great flavor that goes perfectly with Sautéed Balsamic Mushrooms and Onions (page 115).

SERVES 4 / PREP TIME: 5 MINUTES / COOK TIME: 30 MINUTES

1 tablespoon kosher salt

1 tablespoon coarse-ground black pepper

1 teaspoon garlic powder

4 (6- to 8-ounce) New York strip steaks

2 tablespoons olive oil

4 tablespoons Garlic-Rosemary Compound Butter (page 127)

1. Preheat the broiler.
2. In a small bowl, stir together the salt, pepper, and garlic powder.
3. Pat the steaks dry with paper towels, then season both sides with the seasoning mixture.
4. In a large oven-safe skillet, heat the oil over medium-high heat for at least 3 minutes, until very hot.
5. Working in batches, place the steaks in the skillet and pan-sear for 3 to 4 minutes per side. When done, place all the seared steaks in the skillet.
6. Broil the steaks for 5 to 7 minutes for medium-rare, or to your desired doneness.
7. Top each steak with 1 tablespoon of compound butter to melt.

> **PREP TIP:** Prepare the compound butter at least 2 hours before cooking the steak so it has time to set in the refrigerator.

T-BONE STEAK WITH BÉARNAISE SAUCE

Surprisingly tender, this oven-cooked steak is also simple to make. The key to success is ensuring the steak is as dry as possible before cooking. You'll heat it over a very low temperature, apply a reverse sear, then top it with creamy béarnaise.

SERVES 4 / PREP TIME: 5 MINUTES, PLUS 2 HOURS TO SEASON / COOK TIME: 1 HOUR

4 T-bone steaks
1 tablespoon kosher salt
2 teaspoons coarse-ground black pepper
2 tablespoons olive oil
1 recipe Béarnaise Sauce (page 120), warmed

1. Season each steak on both sides with the salt and pepper, then place them on a wire rack set in a roasting pan. Refrigerate, uncovered, for 2 hours.
2. Preheat the oven to 225°F.
3. Place the pan in the oven and roast the steaks for about 50 minutes for medium-rare, or until they are about 15 degrees below your desired doneness.
4. When the steaks are almost done cooking, heat the oil in a a large skillet over high heat for 2 to 3 minutes, until hot.
5. Working in batches, add the steaks to the skillet and pan-sear for 4 to 5 minutes per side. Sear the edges of each steak for about 20 seconds. Remove from the skillet and top with the warm béarnaise.

MIX IT UP: This recipe also works well with filet mignon, New York strip, porterhouse, and rib eye.

PORTERHOUSE STEAK WITH CREAMY PEPPERCORN-MUSHROOM SAUCE

I guarantee this will be the most flavorful porterhouse steak dinner you've ever had. This steak is roasted at high heat, then topped with a savory peppercorn-mushroom sauce. Serve with Twice-Baked Potatoes (page 113).

SERVES 4 / PREP TIME: 25 MINUTES / COOK TIME: 20 MINUTES

FOR THE STEAKS

- 4 porterhouse steaks
- ¼ cup olive oil
- 2 teaspoons kosher salt
- 2 teaspoons coarse-ground black pepper

FOR THE PEPPERCORN-MUSHROOM SAUCE

- 1 (10.5-ounce) can beef consommé
- 1 cup heavy (whipping) cream
- 3 tablespoons salted butter
- 2 garlic cloves, minced
- 1 tablespoon crushed black peppercorns
- ½ cup sliced white mushrooms
- 2 teaspoons all-purpose flour
- Kosher salt
- Coarse-ground black pepper

TO MAKE THE STEAKS

1. Adjust the top oven rack so it is at least 5 inches away from the broiler element. Place an oven-safe skillet on the rack. Turn on the broiler and preheat the skillet for 20 minutes.

2. Coat both sides of each steak with the oil, then season all over with the salt and pepper. Carefully place the steaks in the heated skillet and broil for 3 minutes, then turn the steaks over and broil for another 3 minutes.

3. Switch the oven to bake and set the temperature to 500°F.

4. Insert an oven-safe digital thermometer into the side of one steak and roast for about 5 minutes for medium-rare, or to your desired doneness. Transfer the steaks to a plate and cover them with aluminum foil.

TO MAKE THE PEPPERCORN-MUSHROOM SAUCE

5. Place the skillet over high heat (remember the handle will be hot!), pour in the consommé, and stir to scrape up any browned bits from the bottom. Bring the consommé to a boil and cook for 2 to 3 minutes, until it starts to reduce.

6. Whisk in the cream, butter, peppercorns, and mushrooms. Cook for 1 to 2 minutes, whisking constantly.

7. Whisk in the flour and cook, whisking constantly, for 2 to 3 minutes, until the sauce starts to thicken. Reduce the heat to low and simmer for 1 to 2 minutes. Taste and season the sauce with salt and pepper as needed. Top the steaks with the peppercorn-mushroom sauce and serve.

> **MIX IT UP:** Try this recipe with New York strip, rib eye, sirloin, or T-bone.
>
> **PREP TIP:** If you don't have consommé, use beef broth.

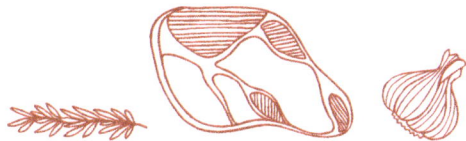

CREAMY CAJUN STEAK BITES

A family favorite, these Cajun steak bites are full of flavor (but not too spicy) and easy to make. Kids love them, too! During a recent sleepover, I made these as an easy meal and my kids not only ate them all but also asked for more! Serve over rice for a full meal.

SERVES 5 OR 6 / PREP TIME: 10 MINUTES / COOK TIME: 35 MINUTES

- 1 tablespoon dark brown sugar
- 1 tablespoon Cajun seasoning
- 2 teaspoons kosher salt
- 2 teaspoons garlic powder
- 2 teaspoons onion powder
- 2 teaspoons chili powder
- ¼ teaspoon cayenne pepper
- 4 (4- to 6-ounce) New York strip steaks, cut into 2-inch cubes
- ¼ cup olive oil, plus more as needed
- 5 garlic cloves, minced
- 1 tablespoon unsalted butter
- ¼ cup heavy (whipping) cream

1. In a large bowl, stir together the brown sugar, Cajun seasoning, salt, garlic powder, onion powder, chili powder, and cayenne. Add the steak cubes and toss to coat well.
2. In a large skillet, heat the oil over medium-high heat. Add the garlic and sauté for 1 minute.
3. Working in batches, add the seasoned steak bites and sear for 3 to 4 minutes per side, adding more oil if the skillet gets dry and becomes smoky between batches. Remove the steak cubes and set aside.
4. Reduce the heat to medium and add the butter to the skillet to melt. Whisk in the heavy cream. Return the steak bites to the skillet and stir well to coat in the sauce.

> **MAKE IT EASIER:** Ask the butcher to cut the steaks into 2-inch cubes.
>
> **MIX IT UP:** Try this with rib eye or sirloin.

BLACK AND BLUE GRILLED STEAK SALAD

This salad is exceptionally flavorful when paired with a lightly seasoned and perfectly seared steak. The blue cheese crumbles and the warm, crispy bacon provide texture, tang, and heartiness.

SERVES 4 / PREP TIME: 20 MINUTES / COOK TIME: 15 MINUTES

2 tablespoons olive oil

8 cups chopped romaine lettuce

½ red onion, sliced

1 cup cherry tomatoes, halved

⅓ cup blue cheese crumbles

12 bacon slices, cooked and chopped

1 cup croutons (optional)

2 (6- to 8-ounce) New York strip steaks

1 teaspoon kosher salt

1 teaspoon coarse-ground black pepper

Blue cheese or ranch dressing, for serving

1. Preheat a grill to high heat (about 400°F), or heat a stovetop grill pan over medium-high heat.

2. In a large bowl, combine the lettuce, onion, tomatoes, blue cheese, bacon, and croutons (if using). Toss to combine. Cover and refrigerate until ready to serve.

3. Coat both sides of each steak with the olive oil and season with the salt and pepper.

4. Place the steaks on the grill and sear for 2 to 3 minutes per side. Lower the grill temperature to medium-low (about 300°F) and grill the steaks, turning once, for another 3 to 5 minutes for medium-rare, or to your desired doneness. Transfer to a plate and let rest for 2 to 3 minutes before slicing.

5. Divide the salad among four plates and top each with sliced steak. Serve with your dressing of choice.

ADVANCED TECHNIQUE: This is also a great recipe to make using the afterburner method (see page 28).

MIX IT UP: Try this recipe with filet mignon, rib eye, or sirloin.

PHILLY CHEESESTEAK SANDWICHES

If you're looking to make restaurant-quality sandwiches in your kitchen, this recipe is for you. Philly cheesesteaks are made with thinly sliced rib eye steak, caramelized onions, and melted provolone cheese. Stuffed into a hoagie roll toasted with garlic-herb butter, these are the most tender, juicy, and delicious Philly cheesesteaks you will ever make! Serve these with my Oven-Baked Steak Fries (page 112).

SERVES 6 / PREP TIME: 20 MINUTES / COOK TIME: 45 MINUTES

- 4 tablespoons olive oil, divided
- 1 large sweet onion, diced
- 4 pounds boneless rib eye steaks, thinly sliced against the grain
- 2 teaspoons kosher salt
- 2 teaspoons coarse-ground black pepper
- 4 tablespoons Garlic-Rosemary Compound Butter (page 127), melted
- 6 hoagie rolls, split
- 6 slices provolone cheese
- 6 tablespoons Smoked Paprika and Garlic Aioli (page 118)

1. In a medium skillet, heat 2 tablespoons of oil over medium heat. Add the onion and sauté for 10 to 12 minutes, until caramelized. Transfer to a small bowl and set aside.

2. Increase the heat to medium-high, add another 1 tablespoon of oil and heat for about 3 minutes, until hot.

3. Working in batches, add the steak slices in a single layer, ensuring there is no overlap, and cook for 3 to 4 minutes. Flip each piece and season with the salt and pepper. Continue to cook until the steak is fully cooked and no longer pink, adding the remaining 1 tablespoon of oil as needed. Transfer the steak to a plate and set aside; reserve the skillet.

4. Using a basting brush, spread the compound butter onto the outside of each hoagie roll, ensuring that all sides are lightly covered.

5. In another skillet, toast the outside of the hoagie rolls over medium heat for about 2 minutes, or until they turn light golden-brown on both sides.

6. Return the steak skillet to medium-high heat. For each sandwich, transfer about ¾ cup of the meat slices to the skillet. Add 2 tablespoons of the caramelized onion and sauté for 30 seconds.

7. Place 1 slice of provolone cheese on the meat mixture to melt.

8. Spread a thin layer of aioli (about 1 tablespoon) on the inside of a toasted roll, then add the meat and cheese. Repeat with the remaining meat, onion, cheese, aioli, and rolls. Serve immediately.

> **MAKE IT EASIER:** For easier slicing, wrap the steak in plastic wrap and freeze for 30 minutes before slicing. Or, even easier, ask your butcher to thinly slice the meat for you.

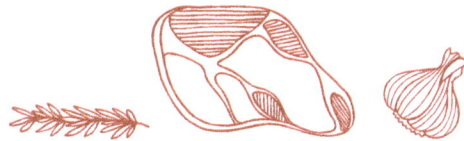

Premium Steaks 57

MONGOLIAN BEEF

Despite the name, Mongolian beef is a dish that originated in Taiwan. I make my version with thinly sliced rib eye. It's my dad's favorite steak dish. The sautéed fresh ginger and garlic puts the flavor meter over the top! Serve this beef over jasmine or basmati rice.

SERVES 6 / PREP TIME: 15 MINUTES / COOK TIME: 20 MINUTES

2 pounds boneless rib eye, sliced ¼ inch thick

3 tablespoons cornstarch

4 tablespoons olive oil, divided

5 garlic cloves, minced

2 tablespoons finely chopped peeled fresh ginger

⅓ cup plus 2 tablespoons soy sauce

⅓ cup water

⅓ cup packed dark brown sugar

¼ teaspoon red pepper flakes

4 to 5 cups bite-size broccoli pieces

1 (5-ounce) can sliced water chestnuts, drained

4 scallions, green and white parts, thinly sliced

1. Put the steak slices in a 1-gallon resealable plastic bag. Add the cornstarch, seal, and shake until the meat is well coated. Set aside.

2. In a small saucepan, heat 2 tablespoons of oil over medium-high heat for 3 to 4 minutes, until very hot. Add the garlic and ginger and sauté for 1 to 2 minutes. Stir in ⅓ cup of soy sauce, the water, brown sugar, and red pepper flakes. Cook for 7 to 10 minutes, stirring frequently, until the sauce starts to thicken. Adjust the heat, if needed.

3. While the sauce cooks, heat the remaining 2 tablespoons of olive oil in a large skillet over medium-high heat for 3 to 4 minutes, until very hot. Working in batches, sauté the steak for 3 to 5 minutes.

4. Add the broccoli and water chestnuts to the skillet with the beef. Cook for 3 to 4 minutes, stirring occasionally, until the broccoli starts to soften.

5. Pour the sauce over the beef and vegetables, along with the remaining 2 tablespoons of soy sauce. Cook for 4 to 5 minutes, until the sauce thickens and the broccoli is tender. Top with the sliced scallions and serve.

> **ADVANCED TECHNIQUE:** If you prefer a thicker sauce, whisk 1½ teaspoons of cornstarch with 1 tablespoon of water until smooth. Stir the slurry into the sauce and increase the heat. Cook until the sauce thickens.
>
> **MIX IT UP:** Try this recipe with flat iron or hanger steak.

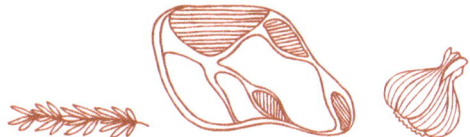

SOUTHWESTERN STEAK STEW

Most people make chili and stew with either ground beef or chuck roast. But I love using a good marbled steak because it adds more flavor. This stew gets a bit of a kick from the picante sauce—don't use salsa. Serve this stew with hot corn bread, over rice or noodles, or topped with shredded cheese or sour cream.

SERVES 5 OR 6 / PREP TIME: 15 MINUTES / COOK TIME: 3 HOURS

- 2 tablespoons olive oil
- 2 pounds boneless rib eye, cut into 2-inch cubes
- ½ yellow onion, diced
- 1 (28-ounce) can petite diced tomatoes, undrained
- 1 (16-ounce) can pinto beans, drained and rinsed
- 1 (16-ounce) can whole kernel corn, drained and rinsed
- 1 cup medium Pace picante sauce
- ¾ cup water
- 1 teaspoon salt
- ½ teaspoon chili powder
- ½ teaspoon ground cumin
- ½ teaspoon garlic powder

1. In a large skillet, heat the oil over medium-high heat for 3 to 4 minutes, until very hot.
2. Sear the steak cubes for 1 to 2 minutes on all sides. Drain the steak on paper towels.
3. Transfer the steak to a large stockpot or Dutch oven and add the onion, tomatoes and their juice, beans, corn, picante sauce, water, salt, chili powder, cumin, and garlic powder. Stir well. Bring the stew to a boil, then reduce the heat to medium-low. Cover the pot and cook, stirring occasionally, for 2 to 3 hours, until the meat is tender and the stew is thickened.

CREAMY STEAK ALFREDO PASTA

Everyone loves a good pasta dish, but adding steak is a game changer. This recipe was inspired by Chef Shawn Melia at the Franklin Chop House, where I used to work. It features thinly sliced rib eye, homemade Alfredo sauce, artichoke hearts, sun-dried tomatoes, and mushrooms served over fettuccine noodles. I go a little heavy on the garlic in the sauce, but that's what gives it so much flavor.

SERVES 6 TO 8 / PREP TIME: 15 MINUTES / COOK TIME: 20 MINUTES

1 pound fettuccine

1 tablespoon olive oil

2 (4- to 6-ounce) boneless rib eye steaks, thinly sliced

8 tablespoons (1 stick) unsalted butter

5 garlic cloves, minced

2 cups heavy (whipping) cream

2 cups freshly grated Parmesan cheese

½ teaspoon kosher salt

¾ teaspoon coarse-ground black pepper

1 (6-ounce) jar artichoke hearts, drained and chopped or halved

1 cup sliced cremini mushrooms

¼ cup oil-packed sun-dried tomatoes, drained

1. Bring a large pot of water to a boil over high heat. Add the fettuccine and cook until al dente according to the package directions. Drain, rinse with cold water, and set aside.

2. Meanwhile, in a large skillet, heat the oil over medium-high heat. Add the steak slices and sauté for 5 to 7 minutes, until cooked through and no longer pink. Transfer to a plate.

3. Add the butter to the same skillet and let it melt over medium heat. Add the garlic and sauté for 1 to 2 minutes. Whisk in the heavy cream and cook, whisking constantly, for 1 to 2 minutes. Slowly whisk in the Parmesan, salt, and pepper. Cook, whisking, for 1 to 2 minutes, then reduce the heat to low. Stir in the artichoke hearts, mushrooms, and sun-dried tomatoes.

4. Add the steak to the Alfredo sauce and simmer over low heat for 3 to 4 minutes. Serve over the fettuccine.

> **ADVANCED TECHNIQUE:** Add ½ cup of sliced black olives and 1 tablespoon of capers for more great flavor.

SOUS VIDE RIB EYE STEAKS WITH SAUTÉED MUSHROOMS AND BALSAMIC VINEGAR SAUCE

If you want a steak cooked consistently at the perfect temperature, sous vide is the way to go. It's particularly great for thick steaks. The temperature of your water bath should be set to the temperature corresponding to your desired doneness (see page 40). So, if you want a medium-rare steak, set the sous vide cooker to 140°F. Topped with a mushroom-balsamic sauce, these steaks are a delicious restaurant-quality dinner at home.

SERVES 4 / PREP TIME: 15 MINUTES / COOK TIME: 1 HOUR

FOR THE STEAKS

- 4 (4- to 6-ounce) boneless rib eye steaks
- 8 teaspoons kosher salt, divided
- 4 teaspoons coarse-ground black pepper
- 4 rosemary sprigs
- 4 thyme sprigs
- 8 garlic cloves, peeled and lightly smashed
- 4 tablespoons olive oil, divided

TO MAKE THE STEAKS

1. Season each steak all over with 1 teaspoon of salt and ½ teaspoon of black pepper.

2. Put 2 steaks in a sous vide cooking pouch or vacuum sealer bag, and top each steak with 1 rosemary sprig, 1 thyme sprig, and 2 garlic cloves. Using a vacuum sealer, seal the bag until all the air is removed. Repeat with the remaining steaks, rosemary and thyme sprigs, and garlic cloves in another bag. Set aside.

3. Fill the sous vide container with about 2 gallons of water. Securely attach the precision cooker to the container. Set the temperature to the desired doneness of the steak and set the timer.

4. Once the water reaches the desired temperature, place the vacuum-sealed bags in the water and cook until the timer sounds.

5. In a large skillet, heat 2 tablespoons of olive oil over high heat.

FOR THE SAUCE

2 tablespoons unsalted butter, divided

4 garlic cloves, minced

1 cup sliced white mushrooms

¼ cup beef broth

¼ cup balsamic vinegar

¼ teaspoon kosher salt

¼ teaspoon ground white pepper

¼ cup heavy (whipping) cream

6. Remove 2 cooked steaks from one bag and sprinkle each steak all over with 1 teaspoon of salt and ½ teaspoon of black pepper. Add the steaks and herbs from the bag to the skillet and sear each side of the steaks for about 30 seconds. Transfer to a plate.

7. Repeat with the remaining 2 tablespoons of oil and remaining 2 steaks, salt, and pepper.

TO MAKE THE SAUCE

8. About 15 minutes before the steaks are ready to come out of the sous vide, heat 1 tablespoon of butter in a medium skillet over medium-high heat. Add the garlic and sauté for 1 to 2 minutes.

9. Add the mushrooms and sauté for 5 to 6 minutes, until most of their juices have released and the mushrooms start to brown.

10. Stir in the broth, vinegar, salt, and white pepper. Turn the heat to medium-low and cook, whisking continually, for 8 to 10 minutes, until the liquid is reduced by half.

11. Turn the heat back up to medium-high and whisk in the heavy cream until it comes to a boil. Reduce the heat to low and simmer for 2 to 3 minutes. Remove the saucepan from the heat.

12. Stir in the remaining 1 tablespoon of butter to combine. Top each steak with sauce and serve.

> **MIX IT UP:** Try this recipe with filet mignon or New York strip steaks.

Premium Steaks

STEAK DIANE

A classic recipe at steak restaurants, this dinner delivers the "wow" factor. This version features a rich and flavorful cream sauce made with mushrooms, garlic, broth, brandy, and cream. Serve the steak with Homestyle Mashed Potatoes (page 114) and a side salad.

SERVES 4 OR 5 / PREP TIME: 15 MINUTES / COOK TIME: 30 MINUTES

- 4 (6- to 8-ounce) filet mignon steaks
- 3 teaspoons kosher salt, divided
- 3 teaspoons coarse-ground black pepper, divided
- 4 tablespoons (½ stick) unsalted butter, divided
- 8 ounces white mushrooms, sliced
- 1 shallot, finely chopped
- 5 garlic cloves, minced
- ⅓ cup brandy
- ⅓ cup heavy (whipping) cream
- ¼ cup beef broth
- 1 teaspoon Dijon mustard
- 1 teaspoon Worcestershire sauce
- 3 rosemary sprigs, leaves removed and chopped, stems discarded

1. Season the steaks all over with 1½ teaspoons of salt and 1½ teaspoons of pepper.
2. In a large skillet, melt 2 tablespoons of butter over medium-high heat. Add the steaks and sear for 3 to 4 minutes per side, searing the edges as well. Remove from the skillet and set aside.
3. Melt the remaining 2 tablespoons of butter in the skillet. Add the mushrooms, shallot, and garlic. Sauté for 5 to 6 minutes, until softened.
4. Carefully pour in the brandy and whisk to combine.
5. Whisk in the heavy cream, broth, mustard, Worcestershire, rosemary, remaining 1½ teaspoons of salt, and remaining 1½ teaspoons of pepper.
6. Add the steaks to the sauce, cover the skillet, and cook for 3 to 5 minutes for medium-rare, or to your desired doneness.

> **MIX IT UP:** Try this with boneless rib eye, New York strip, or sirloin. Cognac or red wine can be used in place of brandy.

OVEN-ROASTED PRIME RIB WITH HORSERADISH SAUCE

This melt-in-your-mouth recipe is made with a rich and savory garlic-rosemary butter and slow-roasted to perfection. Prime rib is a pricey cut of meat, but don't be intimidated. This preparation method is easy. Serve this tender, juicy steak with my Twice-Baked Potatoes (page 113).

SERVES 5 OR 6 / PREP TIME: 5 MINUTES, PLUS 30 MINUTES TO REST / COOK TIME: 35 MINUTES

- 1 (4- to 5-pound) boneless prime rib roast
- 6 garlic cloves, peeled and lightly smashed
- 1 small yellow onion, sliced
- ¼ cup Garlic-Rosemary Compound Butter (page 127), at room temperature
- 1 teaspoon fresh thyme leaves, finely chopped
- 1 tablespoon fresh oregano leaves, finely chopped
- 1 tablespoon kosher salt
- 1 tablespoon coarse-ground black pepper
- Creamy Garlic Horseradish Sauce (page 119), for serving

1. Let the prime rib rest in a dish on the counter for 30 minutes before cooking.
2. Preheat the oven to 450°F.
3. Scatter the garlic and onion slices in the bottom of a roasting pan.
4. In a small bowl, stir together the compound butter, thyme, oregano, salt, and pepper. Cover the entire roast with the butter mixture. Place the prime rib directly on the garlic and onion, fat-side up.
5. Roast for 20 minutes. Reduce the oven temperature to 325°F and continue to roast for 13 to 15 minutes for medium-rare, or to your desired doneness.
6. Remove from the oven and cover the pan with aluminum foil. Let the roast rest for 15 minutes before slicing. Serve with the horseradish sauce.

> **ADVANCED TECHNIQUE:** If your roast doesn't come with a netting, wrap it with netting or cooking twine to hold it securely in place. This also helps maintain heat and pressure during the cooking process, which enhances the meat's flavor.

GARLIC-HERB ROASTED BEEF TENDERLOIN

This beef tenderloin is so tender you can cut it with a butter knife. The secret to making an already incredibly tender steak even more so is to roast it at high heat, then reduce the heat. My Romaine Salad with Garlic and White Wine Vinaigrette (page 117) is a worthy companion.

SERVES 6 TO 8 / PREP TIME: 5 MINUTES / COOK TIME: 35 MINUTES, PLUS 10 MINUTES TO REST

- 4 tablespoons (½ stick) unsalted butter, at room temperature
- 4 garlic cloves, minced
- 1 tablespoon kosher salt
- 2 teaspoons coarse-ground black pepper
- 1 teaspoon dried parsley
- ½ teaspoon dried oregano
- ¼ teaspoon dried thyme
- 1 (2- to 3-pound) beef tenderloin

1. Adjust an oven rack so it is in the top position and preheat the oven to 450°F. Line a rimmed baking sheet with aluminum foil and place a wire rack on the foil.

2. In a small bowl, stir together the butter, garlic, salt, pepper, parsley, oregano, and thyme. Cover the entire beef tenderloin with the butter mixture, ensuring all sides and crevices are covered. Place the tenderloin on the wire rack.

3. Place the baking sheet on the top oven rack and roast for 20 minutes. Lower the oven temperature to 350°F and continue to roast for 12 to 15 minutes for medium-rare, or to your desired doneness.

4. Let the steak rest, loosely covered with foil, for 10 minutes before slicing and serving.

> **ADVANCED TECHNIQUE:** Try the lomo al trapo method (see page 29) to make this next time.
>
> **MAKE IT EASIER:** Use Garlic-Rosemary Compound Butter (page 127) in place of the butter mixture in this recipe.

SLOW COOKER FRENCH DIP SANDWICHES AU JUS

These French dips are slow-cooked with multiple broths and savory herbs that produce the most flavorful beef. By using thinly sliced prime rib, you get a delicious, lusciously tender sandwich. These go well with my Oven-Baked Steak Fries (page 112).

SERVES 6 TO 8 / PREP TIME: 15 MINUTES / COOK TIME: 4 HOURS

3 pounds prime rib, thinly sliced

1 (10.5-ounce) can beef consommé

1 (10.5-ounce) can French onion soup

1½ cups beef broth

1 beef bouillon cube

3 garlic cloves, minced

3 rosemary sprigs

2 thyme sprigs

2 bay leaves

½ teaspoon coarse-ground black pepper

6 hoagie rolls, split

6 slices provolone cheese

1. Put the sliced prime rib in a slow cooker. Pour in the beef consommé, French onion soup, and beef broth and add the bouillon cube, garlic, rosemary, thyme, bay leaves, and pepper. Cover and cook on low for 4 hours.

2. Fill the rolls with meat and top each sandwich with a slice of provolone.

3. Ladle the liquid from the slow cooker into a small bowl for dipping.

> **MAKE IT EASIER:** Ask your butcher to thinly slice the prime rib for you. If you don't have consommé, use additional beef broth.
>
> **MIX IT UP:** Try this recipe with chuck roast or tri-tip. Spread Smoked Paprika and Garlic Aioli (page 118) on the hoagie rolls before filling with the beef and cheese.

Premium Steaks

MONTREAL GRILLED RIB EYE WITH SAUTÉED BALSAMIC MUSHROOMS AND ONIONS

Montreal seasoning is a dry rub made using common pantry ingredients and is delicious on steaks, regardless of how they're cooked. A perfectly seared rib eye steak seasoned with a Montreal dry rub makes a delicious dinner without a lot of fuss.

SERVES 4 / PREP TIME: 15 MINUTES / COOK TIME: 35 MINUTES

2 tablespoons olive oil

1½ tablespoons garlic powder

1½ tablespoons kosher salt

1 tablespoon coarse-ground black pepper

1 tablespoon ground mustard

2 teaspoons dried dill

2 teaspoons smoked paprika

1 teaspoon onion powder

1 teaspoon ground coriander

1 teaspoon red pepper flakes

4 (4- to 6-ounce) boneless rib eye steaks, at room temperature

1 recipe Sautéed Balsamic Mushrooms and Onions (page 115), warmed

1. Preheat a grill to high heat (about 400°F), or heat a grill pan on the stovetop over medium-high heat.

2. In a medium bowl, stir together the garlic powder, salt, black pepper, ground mustard, dill, paprika, onion powder, coriander, and red pepper flakes.

3. Rub the steaks all over with the oil, then coat each steak all over with the dry rub mixture.

4. Place the steaks on the grill and sear each side for 2 to 3 minutes. Lower the grill temperature to medium-low (about 300°F) and grill for 4 to 5 minutes per side for medium-rare, or to your desired doneness. Transfer the steaks to plates and let rest for 2 to 3 minutes. Serve topped with the sautéed mushrooms and onions.

> **ADVANCED TECHNIQUE:** Try cooking these steaks using the over-the-coals method (see page 28).

SLOW COOKER GARLIC-HERB FILET MIGNON AND POTATOES

This flavor-filled filet is one of the easiest you will ever make. It's a perfect choice for a weeknight dinner, and the tenderness in every bite elevates this beyond a meat-and-potatoes dish. Using a slow cooker makes it even easier. Add my Brussels Sprout Salad with Bacon and Balsamic-Dijon Vinaigrette (page 116) for a complete meal.

SERVES 4 / PREP TIME: 15 MINUTES / COOK TIME: 4 HOURS

1½ pounds mini potatoes (such as Gemstone), rinsed

4 (6- to 8-ounce) filet mignon steaks, cut into 2-inch cubes

2 tablespoons olive oil

2 tablespoons unsalted butter, at room temperature

5 garlic cloves, minced

½ teaspoon dried oregano

½ teaspoon dried basil

½ teaspoon dried dill

½ teaspoon kosher salt

¼ teaspoon coarse-ground black pepper

¼ teaspoon Italian seasoning

¼ cup beef broth

1. Combine the potatoes, steak cubes, oil, butter, garlic, oregano, basil, dill, salt, pepper, Italian seasoning, and broth in a slow cooker. Stir until well combined.
2. Cover and cook on low for 4 hours.

MAKE IT EASIER: To keep the steak and potatoes from overcooking, check for doneness at 3½ hours. If you can insert a fork easily into the potatoes, the dish is done.

RED CURRY STEAK AND VEGETABLE KEBABS

This tasty Thai-style recipe features the flavors of a red curry. Serve these steak and veggie skewers over a bed of jasmine rice.

SERVES 4 / PREP TIME: 15 MINUTES, PLUS 4 HOURS TO MARINATE / COOK TIME: 15 MINUTES

½ cup canola oil

½ cup fresh cilantro

¼ cup soy sauce

Juice of 1 lime

5 garlic cloves, peeled

2 tablespoons red curry paste

2 tablespoons oyster sauce

4 teaspoons dark brown sugar

1 tablespoon finely chopped peeled fresh ginger

4 (6- to 8-ounce) New York strip steaks, cut into 2-inch cubes

1 red bell pepper, seeded and cut into 2-inch chunks

1 yellow bell pepper, seeded and cut into 2-inch chunks

1 red onion, quartered

1. In a blender or food processor, combine the oil, cilantro, soy sauce, lime juice, garlic, curry paste, oyster sauce, brown sugar, and ginger. Puree until smooth.
2. Put the steak in a 1-gallon resealable plastic bag and add the marinade, moving the bag around until the marinade coats each piece of steak. Seal the bag and refrigerate for up to 4 hours.
3. Soak 5 or 6 wooden skewers in water for 30 minutes. Remove the skewers from the water.
4. Preheat a grill to medium heat (about 350°F), or heat a grill pan on the stovetop over medium-high heat.
5. Using tongs, remove the steak from the bag and place on a rimmed baking sheet.
6. Pour the marinade into a small saucepan and bring to a boil. Boil for 5 minutes. Reduce the heat to low and simmer for 3 minutes while you prepare the kebabs. Transfer to a small heatproof bowl.
7. To assemble the kebabs, alternate steak, red bell pepper, yellow bell pepper, and red onion on each skewer.

8. Grill the kebabs, turning once halfway through the cooking time and brushing with the cooked marinade several times, for 3 to 5 minutes for medium-rare, or to your desired doneness. Remove and let rest for 3 minutes before serving.

> **MIX IT UP:** Try this recipe with filet mignon, rib eye, or sirloin.
>
> **PREP TIP:** If you're not comfortable heating the marinade used on the raw steak, simply double the recipe and use half to marinate and half to cook with.

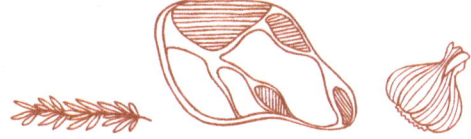

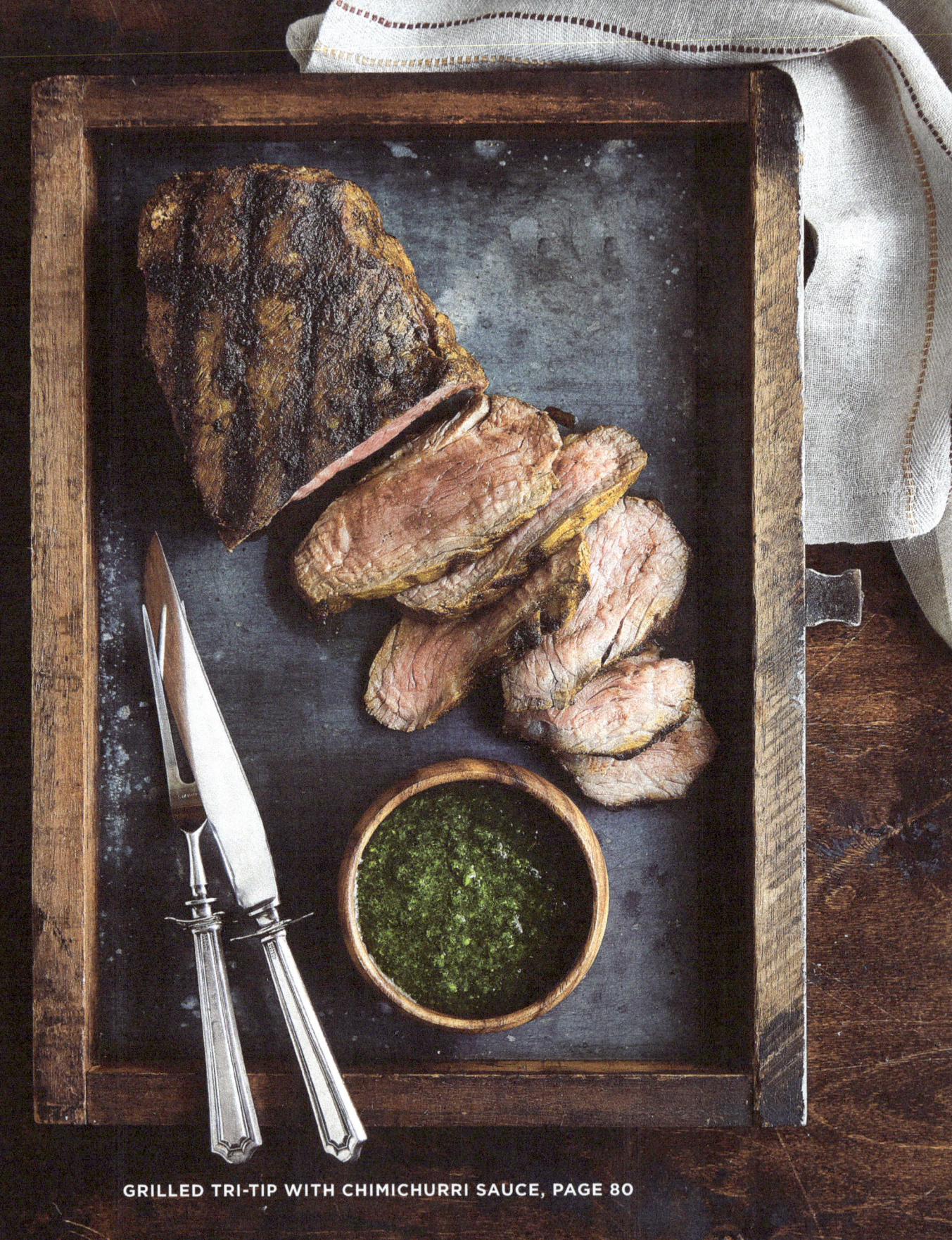

GRILLED TRI-TIP WITH CHIMICHURRI SAUCE, PAGE 80

CHAPTER 6
BUTCHER STEAKS

- **74** Ginger-Soy Sirloin Steak Roll-Ups
- **76** Grilled Flank Steak with Corn-Avocado Salsa
- **78** Cube Steak with Homemade Buttermilk Biscuits and Gravy
- **80** Grilled Tri-Tip with Chimichurri Sauce
- **81** Steak and Broccoli with Ramen Noodles
- **82** Slow Cooker Pepper Steak
- **83** Marinated Flank Steak
- **84** Flat Iron Steak Stir-Fry with Asparagus and Red Pepper
- **86** Spicy Southwest Cocoa-Rubbed Skirt Steak
- **87** London Broil
- **89** Swiss Steak
- **90** Chile-Lime Hanger Steak Tacos
- **91** Classic Beef Stroganoff
- **92** Sweet and Spicy Grilled Hanger Steak
- **93** Chuck Eye Steak with Garlic-Peppercorn Cream Sauce
- **94** Smoked Tri-Tip
- **95** Pressure Cooker Skirt Steak Fajitas

GINGER-SOY SIRLOIN STEAK ROLL-UPS

These flavorful roll-ups make a perfect appetizer, snack, or light lunch and are always a real crowd-pleaser. They are simple to make, low in calories and carbs, and high in protein.

SERVES 5 / PREP TIME: 20 MINUTES, PLUS 4 HOURS 30 MINUTES TO MARINATE AND REST / COOK TIME: 15 MINUTES

FOR THE STEAK AND MARINADE

- ½ cup soy sauce
- ¼ cup packed light brown sugar
- 4 garlic cloves, minced
- 1 tablespoon grated peeled fresh ginger
- 1 teaspoon toasted sesame oil
- 1½ pounds sirloin steak, thinly sliced

FOR THE ROLL-UPS

- 1 tablespoon toasted sesame oil
- 4 garlic cloves, minced
- 20 asparagus spears, woody ends trimmed
- 2 carrots, cut into matchsticks
- 1 zucchini, cut into matchsticks
- ¼ teaspoon kosher salt
- ¼ teaspoon coarse-ground black pepper

TO MAKE THE STEAK AND MARINADE

1. In a large bowl, whisk together the soy sauce, brown sugar, garlic, ginger, and sesame oil.
2. Put the steak in a 1-gallon resealable plastic bag and add the marinade, moving the bag around until the steak is evenly coated. Seal the bag and refrigerate for up to 4 hours.
3. Transfer the steak to a plate and let rest at room temperature for 30 minutes. Reserve the marinade.

TO MAKE THE ROLL-UPS

4. Preheat a grill to medium-high heat (about 350°F), or heat a stovetop grill pan over medium-high heat.
5. In a large skillet, heat the sesame oil over medium-high heat. Add the garlic and sauté for 1 to 2 minutes. Add the asparagus, carrots, and zucchini and sauté for 3 to 4 minutes, until crisp-tender. Season with the salt and pepper. Set aside.

6. Lay a beef slice on a work surface. Place 1 or 2 asparagus spears, some carrots, and some zucchini near one end of the beef slice. Roll the beef around the vegetables and secure with toothpicks. Repeat with the remaining beef and vegetables. Liberally brush the reserved marinade onto each roll-up.

7. Place the roll-ups on the grill, seam-side down, and cook for 3 to 4 minutes per side for medium, or to your desired doneness.

> **MIX IT UP:** Filet mignon or flat iron steak also work well here. Feel free to use any color bell pepper matchsticks in place of, or in addition to, the vegetables called for here.

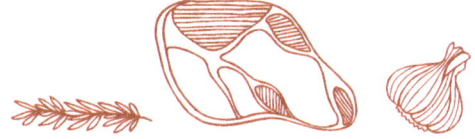

GRILLED FLANK STEAK WITH CORN-AVOCADO SALSA

Fire up the grill for this easy flank steak with garlic-lime marinade. This dish is incredibly flavorful, especially topped with fresh corn-avocado salsa. Both healthy and delicious, this recipe is great to use when making tacos or on its own.

SERVES 6 / PREP TIME: 20 MINUTES, PLUS 4 HOURS TO MARINATE / COOK TIME: 10 MINUTES

FOR THE CORN-AVOCADO SALSA

2 cups corn kernels

1 avocado, pitted, peeled, and diced

½ red bell pepper, seeded and diced

2 tablespoons diced red onion

¼ teaspoon kosher salt

¼ teaspoon coarse-ground black pepper

2 tablespoons extra-virgin olive oil

Juice of 1 lime

1 tablespoon finely chopped fresh cilantro

TO MAKE THE CORN-AVOCADO SALSA

1. In a large bowl, stir together the corn, avocado, bell pepper, onion, salt, pepper, oil, lime juice, and cilantro until well mixed. Cover and refrigerate until ready to serve.

TO MAKE THE STEAK AND MARINADE

2. In a medium bowl, whisk together the soy sauce, lime juice, oil, onion, and garlic.

3. Put the flank steak in a 1-gallon resealable plastic bag. Add the marinade, moving the bag around until the marinade covers the steak. Seal the bag and refrigerate for at least 4 hours, or up to overnight.

4. Preheat a grill to high heat (about 400°F), or heat a grill pan on the stovetop over high heat.

5. Remove the steak from the bag and discard the marinade. Grill the steak for 3 to 4 minutes per side for medium-rare, or to your desired doneness. Remove and let rest for 2 to 3 minutes.

FOR THE STEAK AND MARINADE

2 tablespoons soy sauce

Juice of 1 lime

¼ cup olive oil

½ cup sliced red onion

4 garlic cloves, minced

1 (2-pound) flank steak

6. Thinly slice the steak against the grain. Serve topped with the corn-avocado salsa.

> **MAKE IT EASIER:** Fresh corn cut from the cob makes for the best salsa, but thawed frozen corn works well, too.

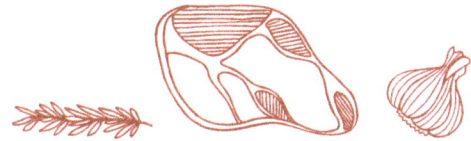

CUBE STEAK WITH HOMEMADE BUTTERMILK BISCUITS AND GRAVY

A Southern-style classic recipe, cube steak and gravy graced our table frequently while I was growing up in Tennessee. The tradition is to serve the steak and gravy over mashed potatoes, but I prefer it on flaky, buttery biscuits.

SERVES 4 / PREP TIME: 30 MINUTES / COOK TIME: 30 MINUTES

FOR THE BISCUITS

- 2¼ cups all-purpose flour, plus more for dusting
- 2 tablespoons baking powder
- 1½ teaspoons kosher salt
- ½ teaspoon baking soda
- 1 cup (2 sticks) salted butter, cut into pea-size pieces
- 1½ cups buttermilk

FOR THE STEAK

- ½ cup all-purpose flour
- ½ teaspoon kosher salt
- ½ coarse-ground black pepper
- 3 tablespoons canola oil
- 4 (4-ounce) cube steaks
- 1 recipe White Country Gravy (page 125), warmed

TO MAKE THE BISCUITS

1. Preheat the oven to 450°F. Line a rimmed baking sheet with parchment paper.

2. In a large bowl, whisk together the flour, baking powder, salt, and baking soda.

3. Add the butter to the dry ingredients, cutting it into the mixture using a pastry blender or a fork. You should see small clumps of butter in the flour mixture.

4. Create a large well in the middle of the ingredients and pour in the buttermilk. Using a fork, lightly mix the flour into the buttermilk until just combined.

5. Dust a clean, flat surface generously with flour. Pour the dough onto the floured surface and fold it in half. Fold the dough several more times until it is lightly covered with flour. Using your hands, spread and pat the dough until it is about 1 inch thick.

6. Using a 2-inch cookie cutter, cut out 8 to 10 biscuits, refolding and forming the dough scraps as necessary. Place the biscuits on the prepared baking sheet side by side, so they lightly touch.

7. Bake for 16 to 18 minutes, until the biscuits are cooked through and lightly browned on top.

TO MAKE THE STEAK

8. In a small bowl, stir together the flour, salt, and pepper. Dredge each steak in the flour mixture until well coated.

9. In a large skillet, heat the oil over medium-high heat. Place the steaks in the skillet and cook for 4 to 5 minutes. Flip and cook on the other for 3 to 4 minutes, until the steaks are no longer pink.

10. For each serving, split 1 biscuit and place a cube steak over the halves. Generously top with the warm gravy.

> **ADVANCED TECHNIQUE:** Don't use a rolling pin to roll out the biscuit dough. Folding the dough by hand results in fluffier biscuits.
>
> **PREP TIP:** Freeze leftover biscuits in a freezer-safe container for up to 3 months. Reheat from frozen at 350°F for 15 to 20 minutes.

GRILLED TRI-TIP WITH CHIMICHURRI SAUCE

A huge crowd-pleaser, this tri-tip is juicy and covered in a flavorful dry rub. This perfectly grilled steak is topped with chimichurri sauce, which pairs well with a variety of meats.

SERVES 5 OR 6 / PREP TIME: 1 HOUR / COOK TIME: 30 MINUTES

2 tablespoons olive oil

1 (2-pound) tri-tip

1 tablespoon kosher salt

½ teaspoon coarse-ground black pepper

½ teaspoon smoked paprika

½ teaspoon chili powder

½ teaspoon ground coriander

¼ teaspoon garlic powder

¼ teaspoon garlic salt

¼ teaspoon onion powder

¼ teaspoon ground turmeric

¼ teaspoon cayenne pepper

¼ teaspoon ground cumin

1 recipe Chimichurri Sauce (page 122), warmed

1. About 1 hour before grilling, remove the steak from the refrigerator and let it come to room temperature.
2. Preheat a grill to high heat (about 400°F).
3. In a small bowl, stir together the salt, black pepper, smoked paprika, chili powder, coriander, garlic powder, garlic salt, onion powder, turmeric, cayenne, and cumin.
4. Rub the oil all over the tri-tip, then cover it with the dry rub.
5. Place the steak on the grill and sear for 2 to 3 minutes per side. Lower the grill temperature to medium-low (about 300°F) and grill the steak, turning once or twice, for 15 to 20 minutes for medium-rare, or to your desired doneness. Remove and let rest for 2 to 3 minutes before slicing. Serve with the warm chimichurri.

> **MIX IT UP:** Try this recipe with hanger, flank, flat iron, or skirt steak.

STEAK AND BROCCOLI WITH RAMEN NOODLES

One of my favorite ways to eat beef and broccoli is over noodles. A staple at Chinese restaurants, this easy stir-fry dish is made even easier with instant ramen. Make this recipe when you need to get dinner on the table quickly.

SERVES 5 OR 6 / PREP TIME: 15 MINUTES / COOK TIME: 30 MINUTES

- 3 (3-ounce) packages ramen noodles, flavor packets discarded
- 1 tablespoon toasted sesame oil
- 1 pound skirt steak, thinly sliced
- 1 cup beef broth
- ¼ cup oyster sauce
- 2 tablespoons soy sauce
- 1 tablespoon finely chopped peeled fresh ginger
- 3 garlic cloves, minced
- 1 tablespoon cornstarch
- 3 cups small broccoli florets
- ½ cup julienned carrots
- 4 scallions, green and white parts, sliced

1. Cook the noodles according to the package directions. Drain and set aside.
2. In a large skillet or wok, heat the oil over medium-high heat. Add the steak and stir-fry for 3 to 5 minutes, until no longer pink. Use tongs to transfer to a plate.
3. Add the broth, oyster sauce, soy sauce, ginger, and garlic to the skillet and whisk to combine. Lower the heat to medium and cook, whisking continually, for 5 minutes. Whisk in the cornstarch and cook, whisking, for 1 to 2 minutes to thicken.
4. Stir in the broccoli and carrots to coat with the sauce. Stir-fry for about 3 minutes, until the broccoli starts to soften.
5. Add the beef to the skillet and mix until all the ingredients are well coated.
6. Divide the noodles into bowls. Top with the beef, vegetables, and sauce and stir to combine. Garnish with the scallions.

> **MIX IT UP:** Try this with flank steak, flat iron steak, hanger steak, or sirloin.

SLOW COOKER PEPPER STEAK

In this easy meal, thinly sliced beef is slow-cooked with onion and sweet bell peppers in a ginger-based sauce. Serve the tender, delicious meat on a bed of cooked rice.

SERVES 4 OR 5 / PREP TIME: 20 / COOK TIME: 4 TO 6 HOURS 15 MINUTES

2 pounds round steak, cut into 2-inch cubes

½ teaspoon kosher salt

1 teaspoon coarse-ground black pepper

1 tablespoon toasted sesame oil

6 garlic cloves, minced

1½ cups beef broth, divided

1 large yellow onion, sliced

1 orange bell pepper, seeded and diced

¼ cup soy sauce

3 tablespoons hoisin sauce

1 tablespoon chopped peeled fresh ginger

1 (8-ounce) can sliced water chestnuts, drained

1. Season the steak cubes all over with the salt and pepper.
2. In a large skillet, heat the oil over medium-high heat for 1 to 2 minutes, until very hot. Add the garlic and sauté for 1 to 2 minutes.
3. Working in batches, cook the beef for 2 to 3 minutes per side. Transfer the cooked beef to a slow cooker.
4. Add ¼ cup of broth to the skillet and stir, scraping up any browned bits stuck to the bottom of the skillet.
5. Add the onion to the skillet and sauté for 2 to 3 minutes, then scrape the contents of the skillet into the cooker.
6. Add the bell pepper, remaining 1¼ cups of broth, soy sauce, hoisin, ginger, and water chestnuts to the cooker. Stir to combine with the beef and onion mixture.
7. Cover and cook on low for 4 to 6 hours.

> **ADVANCED TECHNIQUE:** To thicken the sauce, add 3 tablespoons of cornstarch to the slow cooker, stir, and turn to high about 30 minutes before serving.
>
> **MIX IT UP:** Try this recipe with boneless rib eye, flat iron, sirloin, or tri-tip.

MARINATED FLANK STEAK

This melt-in-your-mouth flank steak recipe features a simple marinade of soy sauce, red wine vinegar, and garlic that puts the flavor over the top. It's perfect for a weeknight dinner or casual cookout.

SERVES 6 / PREP TIME: 10 MINUTES, PLUS 4 HOURS TO MARINATE / COOK TIME: 15 MINUTES

½ cup canola oil

⅓ cup soy sauce

¼ cup red wine vinegar

2 tablespoons freshly squeezed lemon juice

1½ tablespoons Worcestershire sauce

1 tablespoon Dijon mustard

2 garlic cloves, minced

½ teaspoon coarse-ground black pepper

1 (1½-pound) flank steak

1. In a medium bowl, whisk together the oil, soy sauce, vinegar, lemon juice, Worcestershire, mustard, garlic, and pepper.

2. Put the steak in a 1-gallon resealable plastic bag and add the marinade, moving the bag around until the marinade covers the steak. Seal the bag and refrigerate for at least 4 hours, or up to overnight.

3. Preheat a grill to high heat (about 400°F), or heat a stovetop grill pan over high heat.

4. Remove the meat from the bag and let it rest on a plate, uncovered, for 10 minutes. Discard the marinade.

5. Grill the steak for 2 to 3 minutes per side. Lower the grill temperature to medium-low (about 300°F) and grill the steak, turning once, for 3 to 5 minutes for medium-rare, or to your desired doneness. Remove and let rest for 2 to 3 minutes before slicing.

MIX IT UP: Try this recipe with flat iron, hanger, or skirt steak.

FLAT IRON STEAK STIR-FRY WITH ASPARAGUS AND RED PEPPER

Easy and quick, this healthy stir-fry recipe is loaded with fresh vegetables and a delicious sauce made with fresh ginger and garlic. Serve over steamed jasmine rice, ramen noodles, or fried rice.

SERVES 6 / PREP TIME: 20 MINUTES / COOK TIME: 25 MINUTES

FOR THE SAUCE

- 2 teaspoons cornstarch
- 3 tablespoons water
- 3 tablespoons soy sauce
- 1 teaspoon finely chopped peeled fresh ginger
- 1 garlic clove, minced

FOR THE STIR-FRY

- 15 asparagus spears, woody ends trimmed and spears cut into 1-inch pieces
- 3 tablespoons olive oil, divided
- 1 pound flat iron steak, sliced ¼ inch thick
- 1 red bell pepper, seeded and cut into 2-by-¼-inch strips
- 2 cups small broccoli florets
- 1 (8-ounce) can sliced water chestnuts, drained
- 1 scallion, green and white parts, sliced

TO MAKE THE SAUCE

1. In a small bowl, whisk together the cornstarch and water until the cornstarch dissolves. Add the soy sauce, ginger, and garlic and whisk to combine. Set aside.

TO MAKE THE STIR-FRY

2. Pour 2 inches of water into a large skillet or wok and bring to a boil over high heat. Add the asparagus and parboil for 2 minutes. Drain and rinse under cold water.

3. Return the skillet to high heat and heat 1 tablespoon of oil. Add the asparagus and stir-fry for about 2 minutes, until crisp-tender. Transfer to a plate.

4. Heat another 1 tablespoon of oil in the skillet. Working in batches, add the beef and stir-fry for 2 to 3 minutes, until browned but not cooked all the way through. Return all the cooked beef to the skillet and add the bell pepper, broccoli, and water chestnuts. Reduce the heat to medium-high and stir-fry for 3 to 4 minutes, until the vegetables just begin to wilt.

5. Add the sauce and toss to combine. Cook for 1 to 2 minutes, until the sauce thickens.

6. Return the asparagus to the pan and toss to evenly coat in the sauce. Top with the scallion and serve.

> **ADVANCED TECHNIQUE:** Freeze the steak for 15 minutes so it's easier to slice.
>
> **MIX IT UP:** Try this recipe with flank steak, hanger steak, sirloin, or skirt steak.

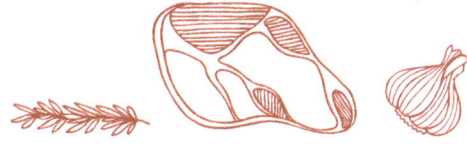

SPICY SOUTHWEST COCOA-RUBBED SKIRT STEAK

I was inspired to make a dry rub that imitates mole sauce with spicy pepper and a hint of cocoa for sweetness. This flavor-packed steak is delicious served on its own, but it also makes excellent tacos.

SERVES 6 TO 8 / PREP TIME: 15 MINUTES / COOK TIME: 10 MINUTES

- 2 tablespoons olive oil
- 2 tablespoons unsweetened cocoa powder
- 2 tablespoons dark brown sugar
- 4 teaspoons kosher salt
- 2 teaspoons ground coriander
- 1 teaspoon chili powder
- 1 teaspoon garlic powder
- 1 teaspoon smoked paprika
- ½ teaspoon ground cloves
- ½ teaspoon cayenne pepper
- ½ teaspoon coarse-ground black pepper
- 1 (2- to 3-pound) skirt steak

1. Preheat a grill to high heat (about 400°F), or place a grill pan on the stovetop over high heat.
2. In a small bowl, stir together the oil, cocoa powder, brown sugar, salt, coriander, chili powder, garlic powder, paprika, cloves, cayenne, and black pepper.
3. Pat the steak dry with paper towels. Rub 3 to 4 tablespoons of the cocoa mixture all over the steak.
4. Grill the steak for 2 to 3 minutes per side. Lower the grill temperature to low (about 250°F) and grill the steak, turning once, for 3 to 4 minutes for medium-rare, or to your desired doneness. Remove and let rest for 3 to 5 minutes, then slice the steak against the grain.

> **ADVANCED TECHNIQUE:** Use a high-quality cocoa powder to enhance the richness and intensity of the dry rub's flavor.

LONDON BROIL

Marinated in beef broth with fresh rosemary and garlic, this steak is incredibly tender and full of flavor. Make sure you serve the meat with several cooked garlic cloves and rosemary leaves—the flavor combination is out-of-this-world delicious. Serve with my Brussels Sprout Salad with Bacon and Balsamic-Dijon Vinaigrette (page 116) or Romaine Salad with Garlic and White Wine Vinaigrette (page 117).

SERVES 6 TO 8 / PREP TIME: 15 MINUTES, PLUS 4 HOURS TO MARINATE / COOK TIME: 1 HOUR 20 MINUTES

3 cups beef broth, divided

½ cup extra-virgin olive oil

⅓ cup soy sauce

¼ cup red wine vinegar

2 tablespoons Dijon mustard

1 tablespoon Worcestershire sauce

Juice of 1 lemon

2 pounds whole top-round steak roast

10 garlic cloves, peeled and lightly smashed

4 rosemary sprigs

1 small yellow onion, sliced

6 tablespoons (¾ stick) unsalted butter, sliced

1. In a small bowl, whisk together 2 cups of broth, oil, soy sauce, vinegar, mustard, Worcestershire, and lemon juice.

2. Put the steak, garlic, and rosemary in a 1-gallon resealable plastic bag. Add the marinade, moving the bag around until the marinade covers the steak. Seal the bag and refrigerate for at least 4 hours, or up to overnight.

3. Preheat the broiler with a rack in the middle position.

4. Scatter the onion slices in a large roasting pan.

5. Remove the steak from the bag and place it on top of the onion slices. Remove the rosemary sprigs and garlic cloves from the bag and scatter them around the steak. Discard the marinade.

6. Pour the remaining 1 cup of broth into the roasting pan.

7. Broil for 10 minutes. Flip the roast and broil for 10 more minutes.

CONTINUED

LONDON BROIL CONTINUED

8. Switch the oven to bake and set the temperature to 450°F. Insert a digital thermometer into the side of the roast and bake for 45 minutes to 1 hour for medium-rare, or to your desired doneness. Remove, cover loosely with aluminum foil, and let rest for 5 to 7 minutes. Slice the beef against the grain.

9. Top each serving with 1 slice of butter, a spoonful of broth from the pan, and a few garlic cloves and rosemary leaves.

> **MIX IT UP:** Try this recipe with flank steak.

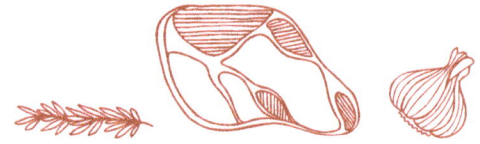

SWISS STEAK

Traditional Swiss steak has a heavy tomato base. My version is a bit more savory, with a beef broth and mushroom base and just a hint of oregano and tomato. Serve over rice, noodles, or Homestyle Mashed Potatoes (page 114).

SERVES 6 / PREP TIME: 20 MINUTES / COOK TIME: 1 HOUR 20 MINUTES

½ cup all-purpose flour

1 teaspoon kosher salt

½ teaspoon coarse-ground black pepper

2 pounds cube steak, thinly sliced

2 tablespoons olive oil, divided

1 shallot, thinly sliced

1 cup sliced white mushrooms

5 garlic cloves, minced

1½ cups beef broth, divided

1 (10-ounce) can cream of mushroom soup

1 (14.5-ounce) can petite diced tomatoes, undrained

1 teaspoon dried oregano

1. Preheat the oven to 350°F.
2. In a small bowl, stir together the flour, salt, and pepper. Coat the steak with the flour mixture.
3. In a large oven-safe skillet with a tight-fitting lid or a Dutch oven, heat 1 tablespoon of oil over medium-high heat. Working in batches, sauté the steak for 2 to 3 minutes per side, until browned. Transfer to a plate.
4. Add the remaining 1 tablespoon of oil to the skillet, along with the shallot, mushrooms, and garlic. Sauté for 30 seconds.
5. Add ½ cup of broth and continue to sauté, stirring to scrape the browned bits from the bottom of the skillet.
6. In a medium bowl, whisk together the remaining 1 cup of broth, mushroom soup, tomatoes with their juices, and oregano. Add the mixture to the skillet and bring to a boil. Cook for 3 to 4 minutes.
7. Nestle the meat into the gravy. Cover the skillet and transfer to the oven.
8. Bake for 1 hour.

> **MIX IT UP:** Try this recipe with bottom round steak.

CHILE-LIME HANGER STEAK TACOS

These are the most delicious grilled steak tacos—I'm talking amazingly good! This minimal-prep recipe starts by marinating steak in a green chile–lime marinade and ends with thinly sliced grilled steak ready to be stuffed into flour tortillas. Serve these tacos with fresh guacamole, pico de gallo, or Corn-Avocado Salsa (page 76).

SERVES 6 / PREP TIME: 10 MINUTES, PLUS 4 HOURS TO MARINATE / COOK TIME: 10 MINUTES

- 1 (4-ounce) can diced green chiles, drained
- ½ cup chopped red onion
- 5 garlic cloves, peeled
- ¼ cup fresh cilantro, chopped
- ¼ cup red wine vinegar
- 3 tablespoons olive oil
- Juice of 2 limes
- 1 tablespoon chili powder
- 2 teaspoons ground cumin
- 2 teaspoons kosher salt
- 2 pounds hanger steak

1. In a blender, combine the green chiles, onion, garlic, cilantro, vinegar, oil, lime juice, chili powder, cumin, and salt. Puree until smooth.

2. Put the hanger steak in a 1-gallon resealable plastic bag. Add the marinade, moving the bag around until the marinade covers the steak. Seal the bag and refrigerate for at least 4 hours, or up to overnight.

3. Preheat a grill to high heat (about 400°F), or place a grill pan on the stovetop over high heat.

4. Remove the steak from the bag and discard the marinade. Grill the steak for 1 to 2 minutes per side. Lower the grill temperature to low (about 250°F) and grill, turning once, for 3 to 5 minutes for medium-rare, or to your desired doneness. Remove and let rest for 3 to 5 minutes, then thinly slice against the grain.

> **MIX IT UP:** Try this recipe with flank steak, flat iron steak, or skirt steak.

CLASSIC BEEF STROGANOFF

A staple dinner loved by many, stroganoff consists of thin slices of sirloin cooked in a creamy mushroom sauce. To keep the dish traditional, serve it over cooked egg noodles.

SERVES 6 / PREP TIME: 15 MINUTES / COOK TIME: 45 MINUTES

- 4 tablespoons (½ stick) unsalted butter, divided
- 1½ pounds top-sirloin steak, thinly sliced
- 4 garlic cloves, chopped
- 1 small yellow onion, finely chopped
- 8 ounces white mushrooms, sliced
- 1 tablespoon all-purpose flour
- 1½ cups beef broth, divided
- ½ cup heavy (whipping) cream
- ¼ cup sour cream
- 1½ teaspoons salt
- ½ teaspoon coarse-ground black pepper
- 2 teaspoons Worcestershire sauce

1. In a large Dutch oven or cast-iron skillet, melt 2 tablespoons of butter over medium-high heat.
2. Working in batches, sauté the steak for 3 to 4 minutes per side, until medium-well. Transfer to a plate.
3. Add the remaining 2 tablespoons of butter to melt. Add the garlic, onion, and mushrooms and sauté for 6 to 8 minutes, until soft.
4. Stir in the flour. Pour in 1 cup of broth, stirring to scrape up any browned bits from the bottom of the pan. Whisk in the cream, reduce the heat to medium, and cook for 3 to 5 minutes, until the sauce starts to thicken.
5. Transfer 2 tablespoons of sauce to a small bowl and stir in the sour cream until well mixed. Stir the sour cream mixture into the pan. Stir in the salt and pepper and cook, stirring, for 1 to 2 minutes, until the sauce is creamy.
6. Return the steak to the pan and stir in the Worcestershire and remaining ½ cup of broth. Reduce the heat to low and cook for 4 to 5 minutes, until the sauce is warm and creamy. Serve immediately.

> **PREP TIP:** Combining the sauce and sour cream separately before adding it to the pot ensures the sour cream won't curdle.

Butcher Steaks

SWEET AND SPICY GRILLED HANGER STEAK

This succulent steak is covered in a dry rub made with chili powder, garlic, cumin, and smoked paprika. It's simple but all you need for a tender and flavorful steak dinner.

SERVES 6 / PREP TIME: 5 MINUTES, PLUS 4 HOURS 30 MINUTES TO MARINATE AND REST / COOK TIME: 10 MINUTES

1 tablespoon chili powder

1 tablespoon garlic powder

1½ teaspoons smoked paprika

1 teaspoon ground cumin

1 teaspoon kosher salt

½ teaspoon coarse-ground black pepper

3 pounds hanger steak

¼ cup Dijon mustard

Sweet and Tangy Steak Sauce (page 123), for serving

1. In a small bowl, stir together the chili powder, garlic powder, smoked paprika, cumin, salt, and pepper.

2. Using a basting brush, coat the steak all over with the mustard. Add the dry rub to the steak, covering both sides fully. Put the steak in a glass baking dish, cover with plastic wrap, and refrigerate for at least 4 hours, or up to overnight.

3. Remove the steak from the refrigerator and let rest on the counter for 30 minutes before grilling.

4. Preheat a grill to high heat (about 400°F), or place a grill pan on the stovetop over high heat.

5. Grill the steak for 1 to 2 minutes on each side. Lower the grill temperature to low (about 250°F) and grill, turning once, for 3 to 5 minutes for medium-rare, or to your desired doneness. Remove and let rest for 3 to 5 minutes, then slice against the grain. Serve with the steak sauce.

> **MIX IT UP:** Try this recipe with flank, flat iron, or skirt steak.

CHUCK EYE STEAK WITH GARLIC-PEPPERCORN CREAM SAUCE

The chuck eye comes from the shoulder, right next to the rib eye, and is very tender, although less expensive. Here it is topped with a savory, garlicky sauce for an impressive dish that takes minimal effort.

SERVES 6 / PREP TIME: 5 MINUTES / COOK TIME: 15 MINUTES

FOR THE STEAK

- 3 tablespoons unsalted butter
- 6 (6-ounce) chuck eye steaks
- 1 tablespoon kosher salt
- 2 teaspoons coarse-ground black pepper

FOR THE GARLIC-PEPPERCORN CREAM SAUCE

- 1 tablespoon unsalted butter
- 6 garlic cloves, minced
- 2 tablespoons all-purpose flour
- 1 cup heavy (whipping) cream
- ½ cup freshly grated Parmesan cheese
- 1 cup beef broth
- 2 ounces cream cheese
- 1½ teaspoons crushed black peppercorns
- ½ teaspoon kosher salt
- ¼ teaspoon smoked paprika
- ¼ teaspoon ground white pepper

TO MAKE THE STEAK

1. Heat a skillet over medium-high heat and add the butter to melt, swirling the skillet to lightly coat the entire bottom.
2. Season the steaks on both sides with the salt and pepper.
3. Working in batches, sear the steaks for 3 to 4 minutes per side for medium-rare, or to your desired doneness. Set aside and cover with foil.

TO MAKE THE GARLIC-PEPPERCORN CREAM SAUCE

4. Reduce the heat under the skillet to medium-low and melt the butter. Add the garlic and sauté for 1 to 2 minutes. Whisk in the flour. Add the cream and Parmesan cheese. Cook, stirring, for 1 minute.
5. Add the broth, cream cheese, peppercorns, salt, paprika, and white pepper. Turn the heat to low and cook, whisking constantly, for 4 to 5 minutes, until the sauce thickens. Top each steak with sauce and serve.

MIX IT UP: Try this recipe with sirloin steak.

PREP TIP: To crush peppercorns, place the whole peppercorns in a small resealable bag and, using a mallet or small pan, pound them until they are crushed.

SMOKED TRI-TIP

Tri-tip becomes even more tender when smoked. Flavorful and juicy, this seasoned steak provides big bold flavors with every bite. Serve with Twice-Baked Potatoes (page 113).

SERVES 6 / PREP TIME: 5 MINUTES / COOK TIME: 2 HOURS

2 tablespoons kosher salt

1 tablespoon coarse-ground black pepper

1 tablespoon garlic powder

2 teaspoons dried minced onion

2 teaspoons dried rosemary

2 teaspoons ground coriander

2 teaspoons dried dill

1 teaspoon red pepper flakes

1 teaspoon ground mustard

1 (2-pound) tri-tip

3 tablespoons olive oil

1. Preheat a smoker to 225°F.
2. In a small bowl, stir together the salt, black pepper, garlic powder, dried onion, rosemary, coriander, dill, red pepper flakes, and ground mustard.
3. Using a basting brush, coat both sides of the steak with the oil, then cover completely with the dry rub.
4. Put the steak directly on the smoker rack and insert a digital thermometer into the thickest part of the steak. Smoke for 2 hours for medium-rare, or to your desired doneness. Remove and let rest for 3 minutes before slicing.

PREP TIP: No smoker? No problem. See page 29 for converting a grill into a smoker.

PRESSURE COOKER SKIRT STEAK FAJITAS

Save yourself time and effort by making steak fajitas in a pressure cooker. A one-pot recipe that has layers of flavor, this staple dish is ready in 35 minutes. Serve with warm flour tortillas, refried beans, fresh avocado, and Corn-Avocado Salsa (page 76).

SERVES 6 / PREP TIME: 10 MINUTES / COOK TIME: 25 MINUTES

2 tablespoons chili powder

2 teaspoons kosher salt

1 teaspoon ground cumin

1 teaspoon garlic powder

¼ teaspoon ground coriander

1½ pounds skirt steak, sliced ¼ inch thick

2 tablespoons olive oil, divided

2 tablespoons sour cream

1 red bell pepper, seeded and thinly sliced

½ yellow onion, thinly sliced

1 (4-ounce) can diced green chiles, drained

¼ cup beef broth

1. In a large bowl, stir together the chili powder, salt, cumin, garlic powder, and coriander.
2. Coat the steak with 1 tablespoon of oil, then toss to coat the steak in the spices.
3. Set your pressure cooker to Sauté mode and add the remaining 1 tablespoon of oil to heat. When the oil is hot, add the steak and sauté for 1 minute.
4. Stir in the sour cream and sauté for 2 minutes.
5. Stir in the red bell pepper, onion, green chiles, and broth.
6. Secure the lid on the pressure cooker and seal the steam valve. Select High Pressure for 10 minutes. When the timer sounds, release the steam and serve.

MIX IT UP: Try this recipe with flat iron or hanger steak.

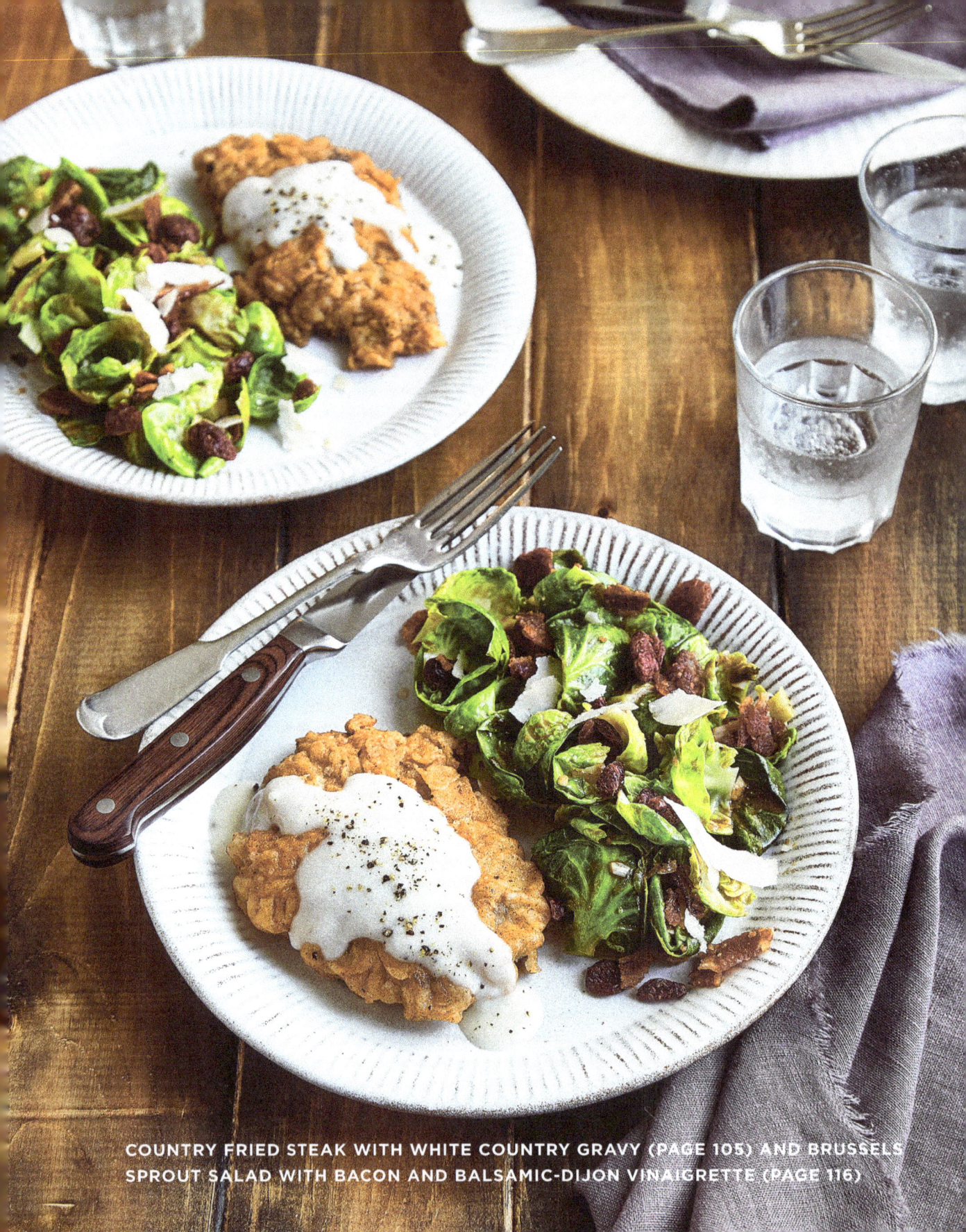

COUNTRY FRIED STEAK WITH WHITE COUNTRY GRAVY (PAGE 105) AND BRUSSELS SPROUT SALAD WITH BACON AND BALSAMIC-DIJON VINAIGRETTE (PAGE 116)

CHAPTER 7
OTHER STEAKS

- **98** Grilled Tofu Steak with Chimichurri Sauce
- **99** Sous Vide Vegan Steak
- **100** Salmon Steak Fillet with Citrus-Cucumber Salsa
- **101** Ahi Tuna with Lemon-Pepper Compound Butter
- **102** IPA-Marinated Grilled Pork Steak with Sweet and Tangy Steak Sauce
- **103** Brown Sugar and Maple-Dijon Ham Steak
- **104** Honey Mustard Ham Steak Panini with Havarti Cheese
- **105** Country Fried Steak with White Country Gravy
- **107** Salisbury Steak with Mushroom Gravy
- **108** Grilled Lamb Chops with Spicy Sesame-Peanut Sauce

GRILLED TOFU STEAK WITH CHIMICHURRI SAUCE

Tofu is an excellent protein-rich choice for a meatless dinner. Marinated in chimichurri sauce, this vegan steak takes on the flavors of cilantro, citrus, garlic, and Italian herbs. Serve with grilled vegetables, Romaine Salad with Garlic and White Wine Vinaigrette (page 117), or Homestyle Mashed Potatoes (page 114).

SERVES 4 / PREP TIME: 20 MINUTES, PLUS 4 HOURS TO MARINATE / COOK TIME: 10 MINUTES

1 pound extra-firm tofu, drained and cut into 8 (⅓-inch-thick) pieces

1 recipe Chimichurri Sauce (page 122)

1. Line a rimmed baking sheet with 3 layers of paper towels. Place the tofu in a single layer on the paper towels, then place 3 more layers of paper towels on top of the tofu. Place a cast-iron skillet (or a baking sheet plus a few cans of tomatoes) on top. Let sit for 10 to 15 minutes to press out excess liquid.

2. Put the pressed tofu in a 1-gallon resealable plastic bag and add the chimichurri sauce, moving the bag around until the sauce covers the tofu. Seal the bag and refrigerate for at least 4 hours, or up to overnight.

3. Preheat a grill to high heat (about 400°F), or heat a stovetop grill pan over medium-high heat.

4. Remove the tofu from the marinade and pour the chimichurri into a small saucepan. Warm the chimichurri over medium heat while you cook the tofu.

5. Grill the tofu, turning often, for about 10 minutes, until firm.

6. Serve topped with the warm chimichurri sauce.

> **PREP TIP:** Add your favorite cut vegetables, such as planks of zucchini, to the marinade. Grill the tofu and vegetables at the same time.

SOUS VIDE VEGAN STEAK

Sous vide offers a simple, foolproof way to cook meatless steak to perfection. Once cooked, reverse-sear the "steak" on the stovetop in hot oil and you'll be ready to serve. These steaks taste delicious served on buns topped with your favorite burger toppings, including my Sweet and Tangy Steak Sauce (page 123).

SERVES 4 TO 6 / PREP TIME: 20 MINUTES / COOK TIME: 1 HOUR 30 MINUTES

FOR THE SEASONING

1 tablespoon kosher salt

1 teaspoon coarse-ground black pepper

1 teaspoon garlic powder

1 teaspoon onion powder

1 teaspoon dried dill

½ teaspoon ground coriander

FOR THE STEAKS

1½ pounds plant-based ground beef

1¼ cups vital wheat gluten

¼ cup water

2 tablespoons white wine vinegar

1 tablespoon toasted sesame oil

2 tablespoons canola oil

TO MAKE THE SEASONING

1. In a small bowl, stir together the salt, pepper, garlic powder, onion powder, dill, and coriander. Set aside.

TO MAKE THE STEAKS

2. In the bowl of a stand mixer fitted with the paddle attachment or in a large bowl using a handheld mixer, combine the plant-based ground beef, wheat gluten, water, vinegar, and sesame oil. Mix on low speed for 1 minute. Transfer the mixture to a work surface and form into a rectangular loaf about ¼ inch thick. Cut the loaf into 4 to 6 strip steaks.

3. Put 2 steaks in each sous vide cooking pouch or vacuum sealer bag. Using a vacuum sealer, seal the bags until all the air is removed. Set aside.

4. Fill the sous vide container with about 2 gallons of water. Firmly attach the precision cooker to the container. Set the temperature to 150°F and set the timer for 1½ hours. Once the water reaches 150°F, place the vacuum-sealed bags in the water and cook until the timer sounds.

5. In a large skillet, heat the canola oil over high heat.

6. Remove the steaks from the bags and evenly coat each steak with the seasoning. Sear each steak for 2 to 3 minutes per side.

SALMON STEAK FILLET WITH CITRUS-CUCUMBER SALSA

This easy pan-seared salmon steak is topped with a light, fresh cucumber salsa for a healthy low-carb dinner.

SERVES 4 / PREP TIME: 15 MINUTES, PLUS 30 MINUTES TO CHILL THE SALSA / COOK TIME: 12 MINUTES

FOR THE CITRUS-CUCUMBER SALSA

- 1 lime, peeled, pith removed, finely diced
- ½ cucumber, diced
- 2 tablespoons minced red onion
- 1 small jalapeño pepper, seeded and diced
- 2 teaspoons finely chopped fresh cilantro
- ½ teaspoon sea salt
- ¼ teaspoon coarse-ground black pepper

FOR THE SALMON STEAK FILLETS

- 1 tablespoon olive oil
- 4 (6-ounce) boneless, skinless salmon fillets
- ½ teaspoon sea salt
- ½ teaspoon coarse-ground black pepper

TO MAKE THE CITRUS-CUCUMBER SALSA

1. In a small bowl, lightly mash the lime with a fork, then stir in the cucumber, red onion, jalapeño, cilantro, salt, and pepper. Cover and chill in the refrigerator for at least 30 minutes.

TO MAKE THE SALMON STEAK FILLETS

2. In a large skillet, heat the oil over medium heat.
3. Season the salmon fillets with the salt and pepper. Pan-sear the salmon for 5 to 6 minutes, until golden brown. Flip and cook for another 5 to 6 minutes, until the flesh is opaque and flakes easily with a fork. Transfer to plates and spoon the cucumber salsa over the top.

ADVANCED TECHNIQUE: If the salmon has the skin attached, pan-sear it, skin-side down, over medium heat and move it around to avoid burning the skin. There's no need to flip it, as the heat will cook the fish through the skin.

MIX IT UP: Try this with sockeye or Atlantic salmon.

AHI TUNA WITH LEMON-PEPPER COMPOUND BUTTER

Making ahi tuna at home has never been easier—or more flavorful. Pan-searing builds flavor and, when you add lemon-pepper butter, you're left with a remarkable main course. Serve over white rice with a side salad.

SERVES 5 OR 6 / PREP TIME: 10 MINUTES / COOK TIME: 9 MINUTES

4 (4- to 6-ounce) tuna steaks, rinsed and patted dry

2 teaspoons Himalayan salt

4 tablespoons olive oil, divided

6 tablespoons Lemon-Pepper Compound Butter (page 33), divided

4 garlic cloves, peeled and lightly smashed

4 rosemary sprigs

1½ lemons, cut into wedges

1. Season the tuna steaks on both sides with the salt.
2. In a large cast-iron skillet, heat 1 tablespoon of olive oil over high heat for about 2 minutes, until hot.
3. Add 4 tablespoons of compound butter to the skillet to melt.
4. Place the tuna steaks in the skillet and scatter the garlic cloves and rosemary sprigs around them. Sear for 2 to 3 minutes, spooning the juices from the skillet over the tuna. Flip the steaks and sear the other side for 2 to 3 minutes, until golden brown and cooked medium-rare. Once you flip the steaks, immediately start taking their temperature with a meat thermometer in the center. Remove the steaks from the skillet at about 10 degrees before your desired doneness. Let the steaks rest on a plate for 1 to 2 minutes.
5. Top each steak with ¾ teaspoon of the remaining compound butter and serve with lemon wedges for squeezing.

> **PREP TIP:** If your tuna steaks are less than 1 inch thick, sear them for only 1 minute per side.

IPA-MARINATED GRILLED PORK STEAK WITH SWEET AND TANGY STEAK SAUCE

A well-crafted India pale ale adds robust flavor to this pork marinade. It's quick to mix and provides a deliciously savory taste after being grilled and topped with my Sweet and Tangy Steak Sauce (page 123). Serve with Twice-Baked Potatoes (page 113).

SERVES 4 / PREP TIME: 10 MINUTES, PLUS 4 HOURS TO MARINATE / COOK TIME: 25 MINUTES

1 cup IPA beer

¼ cup olive oil

4 garlic cloves, minced

2 tablespoons dark brown sugar

1 tablespoon Dijon mustard

1 tablespoon soy sauce

1 tablespoon freshly squeezed lime juice

1 teaspoon coarse-ground black pepper

½ teaspoon ground cumin

½ teaspoon paprika

4 (6- to 8-ounce) pork steaks

Sweet and Tangy Steak Sauce (page 123), for serving

1. In a small bowl, whisk together the beer, oil, garlic, brown sugar, mustard, soy sauce, lime juice, pepper, cumin, and paprika.

2. Put the steaks in a 1-gallon resealable plastic bag. Add the marinade, moving the bag around until the marinade coats the steaks. Seal the bag and refrigerate for at least 4 hours, or up to overnight.

3. Preheat a grill to high heat (about 400°F), or heat a grill pan on the stovetop over high heat.

4. Remove the steaks from the bag and discard the marinade. Grill the steaks for 10 to 12 minutes per side, flipping often, until the internal temperature reaches 145°F. Remove and let rest for 2 to 3 minutes, then serve with the steak sauce.

> **ADVANCED TECHNIQUE:** While the pork marinates, it's important to "massage" the bag occasionally to ensure the marinade covers the entire surface.
>
> **PREP TIP:** Use a British-style bitter IPA or brown ale in the marinade.

BROWN SUGAR AND MAPLE-DIJON HAM STEAK

This ham steak is great for breakfast, lunch, or dinner and it cooks quickly because most ham steak is precooked. The salty-sweet brown sugar glaze is easy to make and is sure to become a family favorite.

SERVES 4 / PREP TIME: 10 MINUTES / COOK TIME: 20 MINUTES

2 tablespoons dark brown sugar

2 tablespoons maple syrup

1 tablespoon Dijon mustard

4 (8-ounce) ham steaks, sliced

2 tablespoons unsalted butter

1. In a small bowl, stir together the brown sugar, maple syrup, and mustard until well combined. Using a basting brush, spread the mixture all over the steaks.

2. In a heavy grill pan or ridged cast-iron skillet, melt the butter over medium-high heat.

3. Working in batches, sear the steaks for 4 to 5 minutes per side, basting frequently with the syrup mixture and butter in the skillet. Serve immediately.

> **MAKE IT EASIER:** Although you can cut individual steaks from a large ham, look for packaged sliced ham steaks at your local grocer.

HONEY MUSTARD HAM STEAK PANINI WITH HAVARTI CHEESE

A panini press is not required to make warm, delicious sandwiches—you can use a ridged cast-iron skillet, a little bit of butter, and pressure to mimic those coveted grill marks panini sandwiches are known for. Creamy melted cheese with salty-sweet ham on a toasted ciabatta roll makes the most delicious lunch or dinner. Serve these with Oven-Baked Steak Fries (page 112).

SERVES 4 / PREP TIME: 10 MINUTES / COOK TIME: 35 MINUTES

FOR THE HONEY MUSTARD

- ¼ cup Dijon mustard
- 2 tablespoons honey
- 2 tablespoons mayonnaise
- 1 tablespoon apple cider vinegar
- ¼ teaspoon smoked paprika

FOR THE PANINI

- 4 tablespoons Garlic-Rosemary Compound Butter (page 127), divided
- 4 ciabatta rolls, split
- 1 (8-ounce) block Havarti cheese, shredded
- 4 thinly sliced ham steaks

TO MAKE THE HONEY MUSTARD

1. In a small bowl, whisk together the mustard, honey, mayonnaise, vinegar, and smoked paprika.

TO MAKE THE PANINI

2. Preheat the oven to 200°F.
3. In a ridged cast-iron skillet, melt 1 tablespoon of compound butter over medium-high heat.
4. Spread 1 tablespoon of honey mustard on the inside of each ciabatta roll.
5. Place 1 roll in the skillet, honey mustard–side up, and scatter ¼ cup of shredded Havarti on top. Place 1 ham steak on the cheese and add another ¼ cup of cheese on top. Cover with the top roll.
6. Using a spatula or a smaller cast-iron skillet, apply pressure to the top of the sandwich and cook for 3 to 4 minutes. Flip the sandwich and apply the same pressure for 3 to 4 minutes more. Transfer to the oven to keep warm. Repeat for the remaining sandwiches, adding more butter before cooking each.

> **MIX IT UP:** Try this dish with sliced turkey and provolone cheese.

COUNTRY FRIED STEAK WITH WHITE COUNTRY GRAVY

I use cube steak to make this cutlet dish, also known as chicken-fried steak. Fried to golden perfection and topped with my White Country Gravy (page 125), this is a comfort food classic that pairs well with Homestyle Mashed Potatoes (page 114).

SERVES 6 / PREP TIME: 20 MINUTES / COOK TIME: 35 MINUTES

1 cup buttermilk
2 large eggs
1½ cups all-purpose flour
3 teaspoons kosher salt, divided
2 teaspoons coarse-ground black pepper, divided
½ teaspoon paprika
½ teaspoon onion powder
½ teaspoon garlic powder
¼ teaspoon cayenne pepper
6 (5-ounce) cube steaks
1 cup canola oil
1 tablespoon unsalted butter
1 recipe White Country Gravy (page 125), warmed

1. In a medium bowl, whisk together the buttermilk and eggs.
2. In another medium bowl, stir together the flour, 1½ teaspoons of salt, 1 teaspoon of black pepper, paprika, onion powder, garlic powder, and cayenne.
3. Season the steaks on both sides with the remaining 1½ teaspoons of salt and remaining 1 teaspoon of pepper.
4. Set up a dredging station with the flour mixture, the milk and egg mixture, and a rimmed baking sheet.
5. One at a time, coat each steak in the flour mixture, then in the egg mixture, and then back in the flour mixture. Place the breaded steak on the baking sheet.
6. Line a large plate with paper towels.
7. In a large skillet, heat the oil over medium-high heat for 3 to 4 minutes, until hot.
8. Add the butter to the oil to melt.

CONTINUED

COUNTRY FRIED STEAK WITH WHITE COUNTRY GRAVY CONTINUED

9. Working in batches, carefully place 2 steaks in the hot oil. Cook for 4 to 5 minutes per side. Transfer to the paper towel–lined plate. Repeat with the remaining steaks. Serve immediately, topped with the warm gravy.

> **ADVANCED TECHNIQUE:** For even more tender results, before dredging the steaks, loosely cover them in plastic wrap and use a mallet or other heavy object, like a rolling pin, to pound them ¼ inch thick.
>
> **MIX IT UP:** Try this recipe with Wagyu center-cut rib eye.

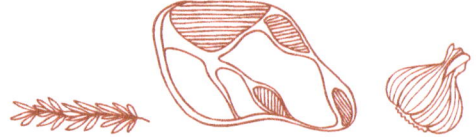

SALISBURY STEAK WITH MUSHROOM GRAVY

In this quick, hearty dinner, juicy beef patties are cooked in a rich, savory mushroom gravy—and a one-skillet recipe means easy cleanup. Serve these mouthwatering steaks with Oven-Baked Steak Fries (page 112).

SERVES 4 / PREP TIME: 15 MINUTES / COOK TIME: 30 MINUTES

FOR THE STEAK

- 1 pound ground beef
- ½ cup bread crumbs
- 1 large egg
- 1 tablespoon Worcestershire sauce
- ½ teaspoon onion powder
- ½ teaspoon kosher salt
- 2 tablespoons olive oil

FOR THE GRAVY

- 2 tablespoons unsalted butter
- 3 tablespoons all-purpose flour
- 1½ cups beef broth
- ¼ cup heavy (whipping) cream
- 1 teaspoon Worcestershire sauce
- 1½ teaspoons kosher salt
- 8 ounces white mushrooms, sliced

TO MAKE THE STEAK

1. In a large bowl, combine the ground beef, bread crumbs, egg, Worcestershire, onion powder, and salt. Using your hands, mix to combine. Shape the beef mixture into 4 (¼-inch-thick) patties.
2. Heat the oil in a large skillet over medium-high heat for at least 3 minutes, until very hot.
3. Add the steaks and pan-sear for 4 to 5 minutes per side. Transfer to a plate, leaving the oil and steak juices in the skillet.

TO MAKE THE GRAVY

4. Add the butter to the same skillet and let it melt over medium-high heat, stirring it into the leftover pan drippings. Whisk in the flour until a paste starts to form.
5. Add the broth, cream, Worcestershire, salt, and mushrooms. Cook, whisking, for 5 to 6 minutes, until the sauce starts to thicken.
6. Return the steaks to the skillet and spoon the gravy over them. Reduce the heat to medium, cover the skillet, and cook for 7 to 8 minutes, until the steaks are well-done and the gravy is thick.

GRILLED LAMB CHOPS WITH SPICY SESAME-PEANUT SAUCE

You often see lamb seasoned with olive oil, rosemary, garlic, and cumin. But I switch things up with this sauce that combines red curry, lime juice, sesame oil, oyster sauce, and peanut butter. A restaurant-quality recipe, this is excellent served over cooked white rice or with my Brussels Sprout Salad with Bacon and Balsamic-Dijon Vinaigrette (page 116).

SERVES 5 OR 6 / PREP TIME: 15 MINUTES, PLUS 4 HOURS TO MARINATE / COOK TIME: 15 MINUTES

3 garlic cloves, minced

¼ cup fresh cilantro

¼ cup creamy peanut butter

2 tablespoons toasted sesame oil

1 tablespoon red curry paste

1 tablespoon freshly squeezed lime juice

1 tablespoon tomato paste

1 tablespoon oyster sauce

1 tablespoon soy sauce

2 teaspoons dark brown sugar

6 to 8 lamb rib chops (about 3 pounds total)

¼ cup water

1. In a food processor, combine the garlic, cilantro, peanut butter, sesame oil, curry paste, lime juice, tomato paste, oyster sauce, soy sauce, and brown sugar. Puree until well combined. Using a basting brush, brush half the sauce all over the lamb chops. Reserve the remaining sauce.

2. Place the lamb chops on a plate or in a small baking dish, cover, and refrigerate for up to 4 hours.

3. Preheat a grill to high heat (about 400°F), or heat a grill pan on the stovetop over medium-high heat.

4. In a saucepan, stir together the reserved sauce and water over medium-low heat until heated through.

5. Place the lamb chops on the grill and sear for 1 to 2 minutes per side. Lower the grill temperature to medium-low (about 300°F) and grill the chops for 5 to 7 minutes more, flipping often, until their internal temperature reaches 145°F. Remove and let rest for 3 minutes.

6. Spoon the warm sauce over the chops and serve.

> **MIX IT UP:** Try this recipe using pork steak with no changes to marinating or cook time.

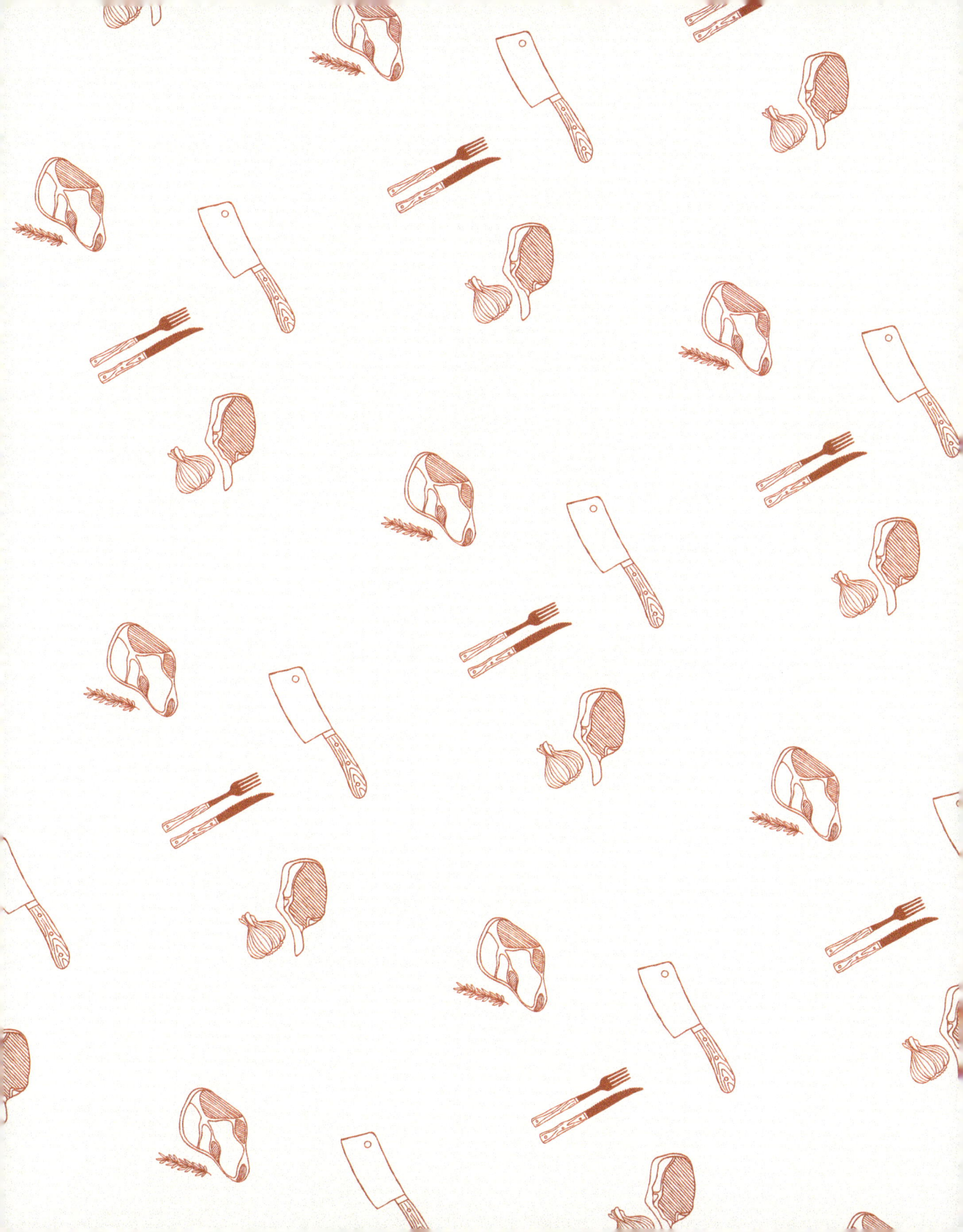

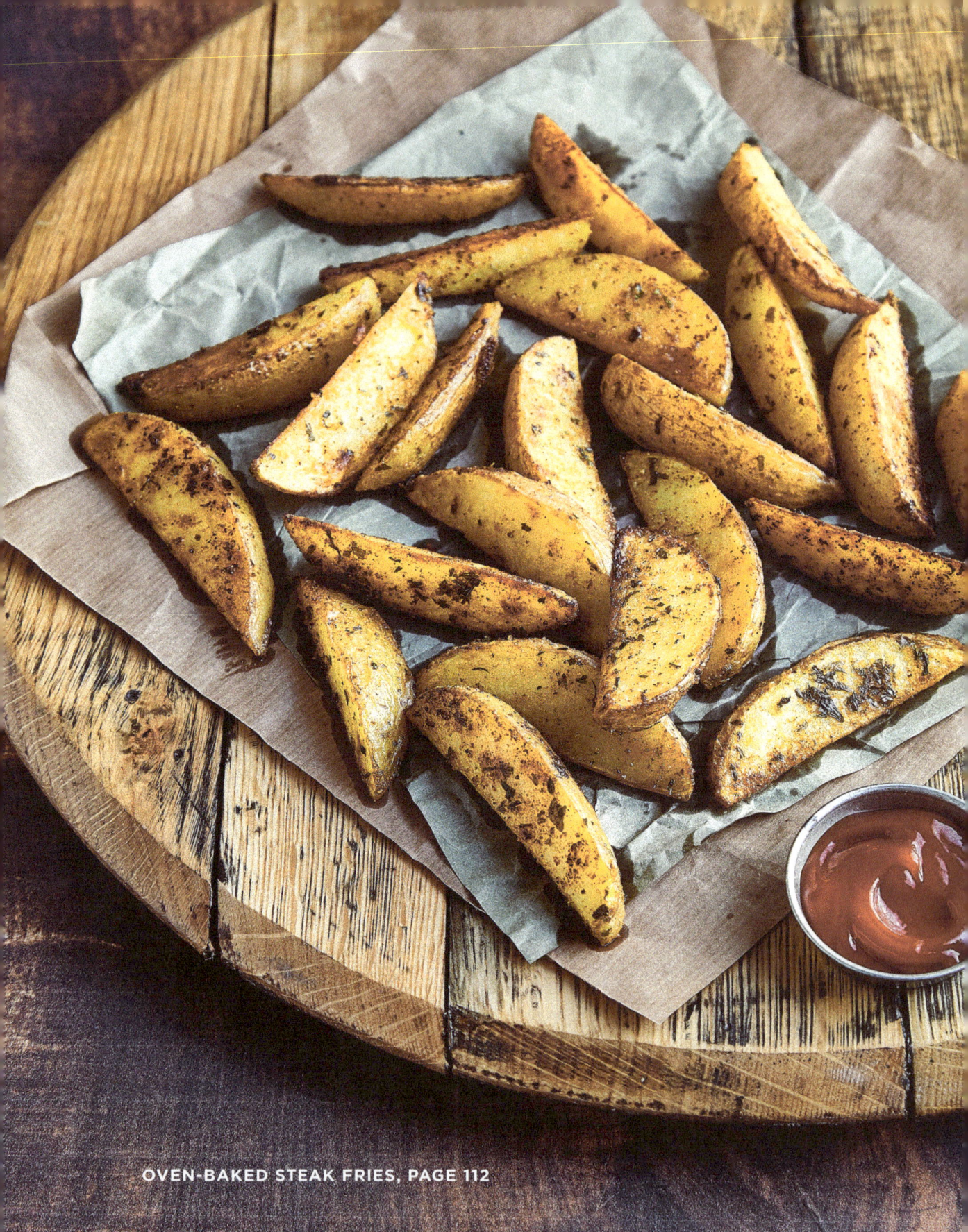

OVEN-BAKED STEAK FRIES, PAGE 112

CHAPTER 8
SIDES AND SAUCES

- **112** Oven-Baked Steak Fries
- **113** Twice-Baked Potatoes
- **114** Homestyle Mashed Potatoes
- **115** Sautéed Balsamic Mushrooms and Onions
- **116** Brussels Sprout Salad with Bacon and Balsamic-Dijon Vinaigrette
- **117** Romaine Salad with Garlic and White Wine Vinaigrette
- **118** Smoked Paprika and Garlic Aioli
- **119** Creamy Garlic Horseradish Sauce
- **120** Béarnaise Sauce
- **122** Chimichurri Sauce
- **123** Sweet and Tangy Steak Sauce
- **124** Smoky Hollandaise Sauce
- **125** White Country Gravy
- **126** Creamy Peppercorn-Mushroom Sauce
- **127** Garlic-Rosemary Compound Butter

OVEN-BAKED STEAK FRIES

Steak fries are the perfect side dish for any steak dinner or sandwich. Baking the fries gives them a velvety soft center with a slightly crispy coating, seasoned with a hint of onion and garlic.

SERVES 6 TO 8 / PREP TIME: 20 MINUTES / COOK TIME: 1 HOUR

6 to 8 large Yukon Gold or russet potatoes, well scrubbed

½ cup olive oil

2 teaspoons seasoned salt (such as Lawry's)

2 teaspoons garlic powder

1 teaspoon paprika

1 teaspoon onion powder

1 teaspoon coarse-ground black pepper

2 teaspoons dried parsley

1. Preheat the oven to 450°F. Line a rimmed baking sheet with parchment paper.

2. Cut the potatoes in half lengthwise, then quarter each half lengthwise. Cut each quarter in half lengthwise to make thin wedges.

3. In a small bowl, stir together the oil, seasoned salt, garlic powder, paprika, onion powder, and pepper. Transfer to a 1-gallon resealable plastic bag and add the potatoes, moving the potatoes around to ensure they are well coated. Spread out the seasoned potatoes in a single layer on the prepared baking sheet. Using a basting brush, spread the remaining coating mix over the potatoes.

4. Bake for 30 minutes. Flip the potatoes and cook for another 25 minutes, or until the fries are golden brown and cooked all the way through.

5. To crisp the potatoes, turn the broiler on high and broil for 3 to 5 minutes. Garnish with the parsley and serve.

> **ADVANCED TECHNIQUE:** When slicing potatoes for steak fries, use the motion of slicing the whole potato front to back and then moving down, pulling the knife through. Chefs use the terminology "tip to heel, then pull."

TWICE-BAKED POTATOES

A classic comfort food, these potatoes are baked, stuffed with your favorite loaded toppings, and baked again, resulting in a creamy, hearty side dish. Though time-consuming, much of the work is hands-off, and these potatoes pair well with any steak dinner.

SERVES 6 TO 8 / PREP TIME: 40 MINUTES / COOK TIME: 1 HOUR 15 MINUTES

3 tablespoons olive oil

3 tablespoons kosher salt, divided

6 to 8 medium russet or Idaho potatoes, well scrubbed

12 bacon slices, cooked and chopped

8 tablespoons (1 stick) salted butter, at room temperature

2 cups shredded Colby Jack cheese

¾ cup sour cream

¼ cup thinly sliced scallion, green parts only

2 teaspoons freshly ground black pepper

1½ cups whole milk

1. Preheat the oven to 450°F. Line a rimmed baking sheet with parchment paper.
2. Generously rub the oil and 2 tablespoons of salt all over the potatoes and place them on the prepared baking sheet.
3. Bake for 45 to 55 minutes, until tender when pierced with a fork.
4. Let the potatoes cool for about 30 minutes. Reserve the parchment-lined baking sheet.
5. Using a small, sharp knife, cut a shallow oval shape around the top of the potato. Using a spoon, gently scoop the potato flesh into a large bowl, leaving ⅛ inch of skin and flesh in the potato shell.
6. Preheat the oven to 350°F.
7. Add the bacon, butter, cheese, sour cream, scallion, remaining 1 tablespoon of salt, pepper, and milk to the potato flesh. Using an electric mixer, or stirring by hand with a large wooden spoon, mix until smooth. Using a large spoon, stuff the potato shells with the mashed potato mixture, slightly overfilling them. Place the stuffed potatoes on the prepared baking sheet.
8. Bake for 20 minutes, or until heated through.

HOMESTYLE MASHED POTATOES

A simple and savory side dish, these velvety mashed potatoes are full of flavor and perfect for any weeknight meal. If you use red potatoes, don't peel them: the peel adds texture and contains all the nutrients.

SERVES 5 OR 6 / PREP TIME: 10 MINUTES / COOK TIME: 20 MINUTES

- 8 red or Yukon Gold potatoes, well scrubbed and cut into 2-inch chunks
- 2 tablespoons unsalted butter
- ¾ cup whole milk, plus more as needed
- 1 teaspoon kosher salt, plus more as needed
- ½ teaspoon freshly ground black pepper, plus more as needed

1. Put the potatoes in a large pot and pour in enough water to cover them by at least ½ inch. Boil the potatoes over high heat for 15 to 20 minutes, until cooked through. Drain the potatoes and transfer to a large bowl.

2. Add the butter, milk, salt, and pepper. Using an electric mixer, mix until smooth and velvety, adding more milk as needed to achieve the desired consistency. Taste and season with more salt and pepper, as needed.

> **MAKE IT EASIER:** Use a handheld masher or a large fork if you don't have an electric mixer.

SAUTÉED BALSAMIC MUSHROOMS AND ONIONS

The perfect pairing for any steak, this recipe features simple ingredients that come together quickly with a rich taste. Try them with London Broil (page 87) and Sweet and Spicy Grilled Hanger Steak (page 92).

SERVES 5 OR 6 / PREP TIME: 10 MINUTES / COOK TIME: 10 MINUTES

- 3 tablespoons unsalted butter
- 5 garlic cloves, minced
- 1 pound white mushrooms, quartered
- 1 large sweet onion, diced
- ¼ cup balsamic vinegar
- 1 tablespoon Worcestershire sauce
- ½ teaspoon kosher salt
- ½ teaspoon freshly ground black pepper

1. In a large skillet, melt the butter over medium-high heat. Add the garlic and sauté for 2 to 3 minutes.
2. Add the mushrooms and onion and sauté for about 5 minutes, until they start to soften.
3. Pour in the vinegar and Worcestershire and season with the salt and pepper. Sauté for 3 to 4 minutes, until the sauce has absorbed most of the vinegar. Serve immediately over your favorite steak.

PREP TIP: To dice the onion, first halve it, then peel it. Lay the onion on a cutting board, cut-side down. Make a series of vertical cuts in the onion half without cutting completely through the root end. Turn the onion and cut crosswise into small pieces.

BRUSSELS SPROUT SALAD WITH BACON AND BALSAMIC-DIJON VINAIGRETTE

This recipe was created by my good friend Tyler, and it is beyond amazing. It's a gourmet-style salad that is a crisp and hearty side dish for any steak. It includes blanched Brussels sprout leaves, bacon, dried cranberries, and freshly shaved Parmesan cheese. Serve this when you're aiming to impress.

SERVES 6 TO 8 / PREP TIME: 20 MINUTES / COOK TIME: 5 MINUTES

FOR THE DRESSING

- ⅔ cup extra-virgin olive oil
- ¼ cup balsamic vinegar
- 1 tablespoon Dijon mustard
- 2 teaspoons minced garlic
- ¼ teaspoon dried parsley
- ¼ teaspoon onion powder
- ¼ teaspoon garlic powder
- ¼ teaspoon salt
- ¼ teaspoon coarse-ground black pepper

FOR THE SALAD

- 1½ pounds Brussels sprouts
- ¼ cup dried cranberries
- ¼ cup finely chopped cooked bacon
- ¼ cup shaved Parmesan cheese

TO MAKE THE DRESSING

1. In a small jar, combine the oil, vinegar, mustard, garlic, parsley, onion powder, garlic powder, salt, and pepper. Cover and shake well; refrigerate until ready for use.

TO MAKE THE SALAD

2. Cut off and discard the Brussels sprout stems. Peel a few layers of the outer leaves, then cut another section of the bottom off and peel another couple of layers. Discard the Brussels sprout hearts. You should have 3 to 4 cups of Brussels sprout leaves. Rinse well.

3. Fill a large bowl with cold water and ice.

4. Fill a medium pot with just enough water to cover the Brussels sprout leaves and bring to a boil. Turn the heat to low. Working in small batches (1 cup at a time), blanch the leaves for 20 to 30 seconds. Using a large slotted spoon or strainer, immediately transfer the leaves to the ice bath for 1 to 2 minutes.

5. Transfer the cooled leaves to a salad spinner or pat dry to remove excess water. Transfer to another large bowl.

6. Add the cranberries and bacon. Shake the dressing well and drizzle it on the salad, then toss to mix. Top with the Parmesan cheese.

ROMAINE SALAD WITH GARLIC AND WHITE WINE VINAIGRETTE

This flavorful salad is made with creamy Havarti cheese and crisp bacon and tossed in a rich, garlic-based white wine vinaigrette. It has the perfect blend of sweet and savory to complement your favorite steak.

SERVES 6 TO 8 / PREP TIME: 15 MINUTES, PLUS 2 HOURS TO CHILL

FOR THE DRESSING

1½ cups canola oil

1 cup white wine vinegar

½ cup plus 2 tablespoons granulated sugar

2 garlic cloves, minced

1 tablespoon kosher salt

FOR THE SALAD

2 heads romaine lettuce, cut into 2-inch pieces

4 ounces creamy Havarti cheese, crumbled

12 bacon slices, cooked and finely chopped

¼ cup unsalted sunflower seeds

¼ cup dried cranberries

TO MAKE THE DRESSING

1. In a small jar, combine the oil, vinegar, sugar, garlic, and salt. Cover and shake well; refrigerate for at least 2 hours.

TO MAKE THE SALAD

2. In a large bowl, combine the lettuce, cheese, bacon, sunflower seeds, and cranberries.

3. Shake the dressing well and drizzle on ¼ cup of the dressing and toss to coat. Add additional dressing, as needed, or serve on the side. (Store any leftover dressing in the refrigerator for up to 1 month.)

SMOKED PAPRIKA AND GARLIC AIOLI

This easy aioli recipe is delicious on leftover tri-tip and roast beef sandwiches, and even on steak tartare. I also like to dip my fries in it! A few simple ingredients, including a subtle kick from smoked paprika, results in an irresistibly smoky, garlicky mayonnaise.

MAKES ABOUT ½ CUP / PREP TIME: 15 MINUTES

6 tablespoons mayonnaise

2 tablespoons extra-virgin olive oil

1 teaspoon freshly squeezed lemon juice

2 garlic cloves, minced

⅛ teaspoon smoked paprika

Coarse ground black pepper

In a small bowl, whisk together the mayonnaise, oil, lemon juice, garlic, and smoked paprika. Taste and season with pepper as needed. Serve immediately, or refrigerate in an airtight container for up to 1 week.

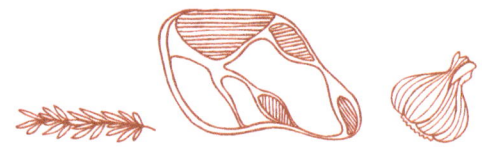

CREAMY GARLIC HORSERADISH SAUCE

I like to tame traditional horseradish a bit with oven-roasted garlic, which provides a subtly sweet flavor with each bite. It's delectable on Ginger-Soy Sirloin Steak Roll-Ups (page 74), Smoked Tri-Tip (page 94), and, of course, Oven-Roasted Prime Rib with Horseradish Sauce (page 65).

MAKES ABOUT 1 CUP / PREP TIME: 10 MINUTES, PLUS 3 HOURS TO CHILL / COOK TIME: 45 MINUTES

1 small head garlic

1¼ teaspoons kosher salt, divided

2 teaspoons olive oil

½ cup sour cream

½ cup prepared horseradish

½ teaspoon freshly squeezed lemon juice

¼ teaspoon Worcestershire sauce

¼ teaspoon ground white pepper

1. Preheat the oven to 400°F.
2. Cut the top off the garlic head so the cloves are exposed. Sprinkle with ¼ teaspoon of salt and drizzle the oil over the garlic. Wrap the garlic in aluminum foil and place it in a small baking dish or oven-safe skillet.
3. Bake for 45 minutes. Let cool.
4. Unwrap the garlic head and gently remove the individual cloves from their skins. Finely chop.
5. In a small bowl, stir together the chopped garlic, sour cream, horseradish, lemon juice, Worcestershire, and white pepper. Cover and refrigerate for at least 3 hours before serving.

BÉARNAISE SAUCE

This classic sauce originated in France and is similar to hollandaise, except it includes shallot, peppercorns, and fresh tarragon for additional layers of flavor. The key to getting the right consistency is keeping the egg yolks and butter warm. This sauce pairs especially well with my Pan-Seared New York Strip with Garlic-Rosemary Compound Butter (page 50) and Garlic-Herb Roasted Beef Tenderloin (page 66), as well as poached eggs and roasted vegetables.

MAKES ABOUT 1½ CUPS / PREP TIME: 5 MINUTES / COOK TIME: 25 MINUTES

1 tablespoon plus 1 cup (2 sticks) unsalted butter

1 shallot, finely chopped

1 garlic clove, chopped

½ teaspoon kosher salt

1 tablespoon whole black peppercorns

¼ cup Chardonnay

2 tablespoons white wine vinegar

4 large egg yolks, at room temperature

1 tablespoon freshly squeezed lemon juice

1 tablespoon warm water

2 tablespoons finely chopped fresh tarragon

¼ teaspoon paprika

⅛ teaspoon ground white pepper

1. In a small saucepan, melt 1 tablespoon of butter over medium heat. Stir in the shallot, garlic, salt, and peppercorns. Reduce the heat to medium-low and slowly stir in the Chardonnay and vinegar. Cook, stirring, for 1 to 2 minutes.

2. Turn the heat to medium-high and bring the liquid to a boil. Cook for 5 to 6 minutes, whisking occasionally, until the mixture has thickened and reduced to about 2 tablespoons.

3. Using a fine-mesh strainer, carefully strain the liquid into a small bowl, pressing down on the solids to extract as much liquid as possible. Set aside to cool completely.

4. While the mixture cools, fill a blender with very hot water to warm it.

5. Wipe out the saucepan and return it to medium heat. Melt the remaining 1 cup of butter until the butter starts to foam. Transfer the butter to a glass measuring cup.

6. Pour out the water from the blender and dry it with paper towels.

7. In the blender, combine the egg yolks, lemon juice, and warm water. Puree until smooth.

8. Remove the center cap from the lid and, with the blender running, slowly pour in the hot butter. Continue blending for 2 to 3 minutes, until the liquid thickens and is creamy. Pour the sauce into a medium bowl.

9. Whisk in the wine reduction, tarragon, paprika, and white pepper. Serve immediately. The longer it sits, the more it will lose its smooth, thick texture.

> **ADVANCED TECHNIQUE:** Béarnaise sauce cannot be cooled and reheated. To keep the sauce warm while finishing other dishes, pour about 1 cup of water into a large pot and bring to a low boil. Turn off the heat. Transfer the sauce to a large glass bowl. Place the bowl in the pot of water to keep warm for up to 30 minutes.
>
> **MAKE IT EASIER:** To quicken the cooling process in step 3, refrigerate the mixture for 7 to 10 minutes.

CHIMICHURRI SAUCE

This sauce, which originated in Argentina, has a robust flavor and pairs well with just about any type of meat, but particularly steak, like my Garlic-Herb Roasted Beef Tenderloin (page 66). With a quick prep that makes the food processor do all the work, this also doubles as a marinade for steak or tofu.

MAKES ABOUT ¾ CUP / PREP TIME: 10 MINUTES / COOK TIME: 5 MINUTES

3 garlic cloves, peeled
½ small shallot, peeled
½ cup fresh parsley leaves
½ cup fresh cilantro leaves
1 tablespoon fresh oregano leaves
1 teaspoon kosher salt
¼ teaspoon freshly ground black pepper
½ teaspoon ground cumin
2 tablespoons red wine vinegar
Juice of ½ lime
½ cup olive oil

1. In a food processor, combine the garlic, shallot, parsley, cilantro, oregano, salt, pepper, and cumin and blend until mostly smooth. With the processor running, slowly add the vinegar, lime juice, and oil. Blend until well combined.

2. Transfer the chimichurri to a small saucepan and place it over medium-low heat for 5 minutes to warm before serving.

3. Refrigerate leftovers in an airtight container for up to 2 weeks.

SWEET AND TANGY STEAK SAUCE

If you like steak sauce, you'll love this sweet and tangy version. This sauce reminds me of a combination of ketchup and A.1. Sauce and pairs well with just about any steak, like my Sous Vide Vegan Steak (page 99) or Marinated Flank Steak (page 83).

MAKES ABOUT 1½ CUPS / PREP TIME: 5 MINUTES / COOK TIME: 25 MINUTES

Juice of ½ orange
½ cup balsamic vinegar
½ cup Worcestershire sauce
¼ cup Dijon mustard
3 tablespoons tomato paste
3 garlic cloves, minced
2 teaspoons dark brown sugar
1½ tablespoons dried minced onion
½ teaspoon celery seed
½ teaspoon kosher salt
½ teaspoon coarse-ground black pepper
¼ cup golden raisins

1. In a medium saucepan, whisk together the orange juice, vinegar, Worcestershire, mustard, tomato paste, garlic, brown sugar, dried onion, celery seed, salt, and pepper. Stir in the raisins. Bring to a boil over high heat, then reduce the heat to low, cover, and simmer the sauce for 20 minutes.

2. Carefully transfer the sauce to a blender or food processor and puree until smooth.

3. Let completely cool, then refrigerate in an airtight container for up to 1 week.

PREP TIP: If your sauce is too thick to puree, add ¼ cup of water.

SMOKY HOLLANDAISE SAUCE

Hollandaise sauce is not as "finicky" as Béarnaise Sauce (page 120), but you do have to keep the butter hot the entire time you're preparing it. My version of this famous sauce is seasoned with cayenne, white pepper, and a hint of smoked paprika. This sauce tastes great on steak, like my Marinated Flank Steak (page 83), Pan-Seared New York Strip with Garlic-Rosemary Compound Butter (page 50), or Garlic-Herb Roasted Beef Tenderloin (page 66), as well as on poached salmon, asparagus, and the classic eggs Benedict.

MAKES ABOUT ¾ CUP / PREP TIME: 5 MINUTES / COOK TIME: 20 MINUTES

8 tablespoons (1 stick) unsalted butter

3 large egg yolks

1 tablespoon freshly squeezed lemon juice

¼ teaspoon kosher salt

⅛ teaspoon cayenne pepper

⅛ teaspoon ground white pepper

⅛ teaspoon smoked paprika

1. In a small saucepan, melt the butter over medium-high heat for 1 to 2 minutes, until it starts to lightly foam and is very hot.

2. In a blender, combine the egg yolks, lemon juice, and salt and blend for about 10 seconds, until well combined. Remove the center cap from the lid and, with the blender running, slowly pour in the hot butter and blend for 1 to 2 minutes, until the sauce starts to thicken. Transfer to a small bowl.

3. Whisk in the cayenne, white pepper, and paprika until well combined. Serve warm.

> **PREP TIP:** The sauce will not properly emulsify unless the butter is very hot, not just melted. Heat the butter on the stovetop to manage the heat properly.

WHITE COUNTRY GRAVY

I learned to make this gravy while growing up in the country in Tennessee, hence the name "country gravy." This is my go-to gravy for Country Fried Steak (page 105), Cube Steak with Homemade Buttermilk Biscuits (page 78), and Homestyle Mashed Potatoes (page 114).

MAKES ABOUT 1½ CUPS / PREP TIME: 5 MINUTES / COOK TIME: 20 MINUTES

- 3 tablespoons bacon grease or other grease from cooked meat
- ¼ cup all-purpose flour
- 1 cup whole milk
- ½ cup buttermilk
- ¼ teaspoon kosher salt, plus more as needed
- ¼ teaspoon coarse-ground black pepper, plus more as needed

1. In a medium skillet, heat the grease over medium-high heat. Whisk in the flour until a thick paste forms.
2. Slowly whisk in the milk and buttermilk.
3. Whisk in the salt and pepper until the clumps are smaller in size.
4. Lower the heat to medium and cook the gravy, whisking, for 2 to 3 minutes, until it thickens. Taste and season with additional salt and pepper, as needed. Clumps are okay but should be small. Serve immediately.

> **PREP TIP:** If you have saved leftover grease from meat you've cooked, like bacon, use it here. Otherwise, use the remaining grease in the pan after you make country fried steak or cube steak. Butter can be used as well, but it will be less flavorful.

CREAMY PEPPERCORN-MUSHROOM SAUCE

Every time I make steak, my family asks if I'm serving it with this sauce—that's how rich and flavorful it is. Try it with my Pan-Seared Filet Mignon (page 37), Sous Vide New York Strip Steak (page 41), or Garlic-Herb Roasted Beef Tenderloin (page 66). A steakhouse classic, this sauce is also delicious on other cuts of meat and vegetables.

MAKES ABOUT 2 CUPS / PREP TIME: 5 MINUTES / COOK TIME: 10 MINUTES

- 3 tablespoons bacon grease or other grease from cooked meat
- 1 (10.5-ounce) can beef consommé
- 3 tablespoons salted butter
- 1 cup heavy (whipping) cream
- 2 garlic cloves, minced
- 1 tablespoon freshly ground black pepper, plus more as needed
- ½ cup sliced white mushrooms
- 2 teaspoons all-purpose flour
- Kosher salt

1. In a medium skillet, heat the grease over medium-high heat. Add the consommé and bring to a boil. Cook for 2 to 3 minutes, until it starts to reduce.

2. Whisk in the butter, heavy cream, garlic, pepper, and mushrooms and cook for 1 to 2 minutes.

3. Add the flour and cook, whisking, for 2 to 3 minutes, until the sauce starts to thicken. Reduce the heat to low and simmer the sauce for 1 to 2 minutes. Taste and season with salt and pepper, as needed.

> **ADVANCED TECHNIQUE:** If you're making this sauce after pan-searing steak, add the beef consommé to the pan and use a spatula to scrape the bottom of the skillet to loosen any browned bits.
>
> **MAKE IT EASIER:** If you don't have leftover grease from cooked meat, use unsalted butter. If you don't have consommé, use beef broth.

GARLIC-ROSEMARY COMPOUND BUTTER

By blending simple ingredients into softened butter, you can easily create a variety of flavors. Fresh garlic and rosemary is one of my favorite flavor combinations. It works well with seared steak, like my Pan-Seared Filet Mignon (page 37), Sous Vide New York Strip Steak (page 41), or Garlic-Rosemary Filet Mignon (page 30). It's also great on garlic bread and on steamed or grilled vegetables.

MAKES ABOUT 1 CUP / PREP TIME: 10 MINUTES, PLUS 2 HOURS TO CHILL

- 1 cup (2 sticks) unsalted butter, at room temperature
- 6 garlic cloves, minced
- 2 rosemary sprigs, leaves removed and chopped, stems discarded
- ¾ teaspoon kosher salt
- ¼ teaspoon coarse-ground black pepper

1. In a medium bowl, combine the butter, garlic, rosemary, salt, and pepper. Using an electric mixer, mix on low speed until well combined. (Alternatively, you can use a handheld whisk.)

2. Transfer the butter to a small piece of parchment paper. Starting from one edge of the parchment, carefully roll the butter to form a log, then twist the ends of the parchment on both sides to seal.

3. Refrigerate for at least 2 hours. Store leftovers in a resealable bag or airtight container in the fridge for up to 2 weeks.

> **ADVANCED TECHNIQUE:** Use your favorite fresh herbs in this recipe, such as thyme, tarragon, and basil.

Sides and Sauces

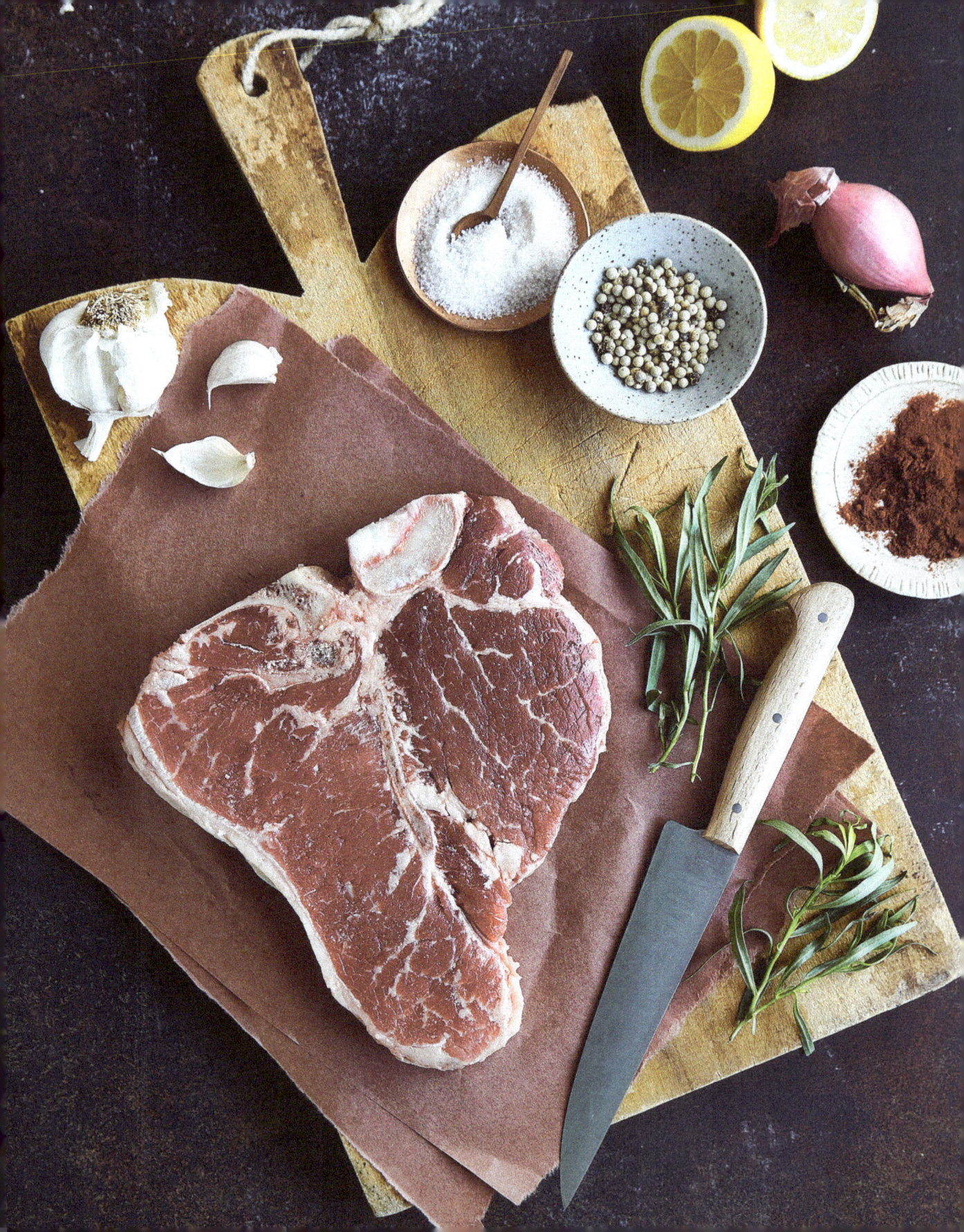

Measurement Conversions

VOLUME EQUIVALENTS (LIQUID)

US Standard	US Standard (ounces)	Metric (approximate)
2 tablespoons	1 fl. oz.	30 mL
¼ cup	2 fl. oz.	60 mL
½ cup	4 fl. oz.	120 mL
1 cup	8 fl. oz.	240 mL
1½ cups	12 fl. oz.	355 mL
2 cups or 1 pint	16 fl. oz.	475 mL
4 cups or 1 quart	32 fl. oz.	1 L
1 gallon	128 fl. oz.	4 L

OVEN TEMPERATURES

Fahrenheit (F)	Celsius (C) (approximate)
250°F	120°C
300°F	150°C
325°F	165°C
350°F	180°C
375°F	190°C
400°F	200°C
425°F	220°C
450°F	230°C

VOLUME EQUIVALENTS (DRY)

US Standard	Metric (approximate)
⅛ teaspoon	0.5 mL
¼ teaspoon	1 mL
½ teaspoon	2 mL
¾ teaspoon	4 mL
1 teaspoon	5 mL
1 tablespoon	15 mL
¼ cup	59 mL
⅓ cup	79 mL
½ cup	118 mL
⅔ cup	156 mL
¾ cup	177 mL
1 cup	235 mL
2 cups or 1 pint	475 mL
3 cups	700 mL
4 cups or 1 quart	1 L

WEIGHT EQUIVALENTS

US Standard	Metric (approximate)
½ ounce	15 g
1 ounce	30 g
2 ounces	60 g
4 ounces	115 g
8 ounces	225 g
12 ounces	340 g
16 ounces or 1 pound	455 g

Index

A

Ahi Tuna with Lemon-Pepper Compound Butter, 101
    Aioli, Smoked Paprika and Garlic, 118
Aluminum foil, 18
Artichoke hearts
    Creamy Steak Alfredo Pasta, 61
Asparagus
    Flat Iron Steak Stir-Fry with Asparagus and Red Pepper, 84–85
    Ginger-Soy Sirloin Steak Roll-Ups, 74–75
Avocado-Corn Salsa, 76

B

Bacon
    Black and Blue Grilled Steak Salad, 55
    Brussels Sprout Salad with Bacon and Balsamic-Dijon Vinaigrette, 116
    Romaine Salad with Garlic and White Wine Vinaigrette, 117
    Twice-Baked Potatoes, 113
Baking sheets, 18
Basting brushes, 18
Beans
    Southwestern Steak Stew, 60
Béarnaise Sauce, 120–121
Beef quality grades, 17
Beef steaks. *See* Steak; *specific types of steak*
Biscuits, Homemade Buttermilk, and Gravy, Cube Steak with, 78–79
Black and Blue Grilled Steak Salad, 55
Black Angus, 16
Brining steaks, 21
Broccoli
    Flat Iron Steak Stir-Fry with Asparagus and Red Pepper, 84–85
    Mongolian Beef, 58–59
    Steak and Broccoli with Ramen Noodles, 81
Broiling steak, 36
Brown sugar
    Brown Sugar and Maple Dijon Ham Steak, 103
    light and dark, for recipes, 20
Brussels Sprout Salad with Bacon and Balsamic-Dijon Vinaigrette, 116
Butter
    Garlic-Rosemary Compound Butter, 127
    Lemon-Pepper Compound Butter, 33
    salted and unsalted, for recipes, 20

C

Cajun Steak Bites, Creamy, 54
Carrots
    Ginger-Soy Sirloin Steak Roll-Ups, 74–75
    Steak and Broccoli with Ramen Noodles, 81
Cast-iron skillet, 18
Certified Black Angus, 16
Charcoal grills
    building fire in, 28

   searing meat on, 28
   turning into a smoker, 29
Cheese
   Black and Blue Grilled Steak Salad, 55
   Creamy Steak Alfredo Pasta, 61
   Garlic-Peppercorn Cream Sauce, 93
   Honey Mustard Ham Steak Panini with Havarti Cheese, 104
   Philly Cheesesteak Sandwiches, 56–57
   Romaine Salad with Garlic and White Wine Vinaigrette, 117
   Slow Cooker French Dip Sandwiches au Jus, 67
   Twice-Baked Potatoes, 113
Chef's knife, 18
Chile peppers
   Chile-Lime Hanger Steak Tacos, 90
   Citrus-Cucumber Salsa, 100
   Pressure Cooker Skirt Steak Fajitas, 95
Chimichurri Sauce, 122
Choice grade, 17
Chuck Eye Steak with Garlic-Peppercorn Cream Sauce, 93
Citrus-Cucumber Salsa, 100
Classic Beef Stroganoff, 91
Cocoa-Rubbed Skirt Steak, Spicy Southwest, 86
Compound butter
   Garlic-Rosemary Compound Butter, 127
   Lemon-Pepper Compound Butter, 33
Corn
   Corn-Avocado Salsa, 76
   Southwestern Steak Stew, 60
Country Fried Steak with White Country Gravy, 105–106
Cream Sauce, Garlic Peppercorn, 93

Creamy Cajun Steak Bites, 54
Creamy Garlic Horseradish Sauce, 119
Creamy Peppercorn-Mushroom Sauce, 126
Creamy Steak Alfredo Pasta, 61
Cube steak
   Country Fried Steak with White Country Gravy, 105–106
   Cube Steak with Homemade Buttermilk Biscuits and Gravy, 78–79
   Swiss Steak, 89
Cucumber-Citrus Salsa, 100
Cutting boards, 18

D

Deep-Fried Boneless Rib Eye, 43
Deep fryer, 19
Deep-frying steak, 42
Digital meat thermometer, 18
Dijon-Maple and Brown Sugar Ham Steak, 103
Dry aging process, 16

F

Fajitas, Pressure Cooker Skirt Steak, 95
Fat, trimming, 21
Filet mignon
  about, 7
  Garlic-Herb Roasted Beef Tenderloin, 66
  Garlic-Rosemary Filet Mignon, 30–31
  Pan-Seared Filet Mignon, 37
  Slow Cooker Garlic-Herb Filet Mignon and Potatoes, 69
  Steak Diane, 64
  Steak Tartare, 45

Fish
  Ahi Tuna with Lemon-Pepper Compound Butter, 101
  Salmon Steak Fillet with Citrus-Cucumber Salsa, 100
Flank steak
  about, 9
  Grilled Flank Steak with Corn-Avocado Salsa, 76–77
  Marinated Flank Steak, 83
Flat iron steak
  about, 9
  Flat Iron Steak Stir-Fry with Asparagus and Red Pepper, 84–85
Foil aluminum, 18
French Dip Sandwiches au Jus, Slow Cooker, 67
Fries, Steak, Oven-Baked, 112

G

Garlic
  Creamy Garlic Horseradish Sauce, 119
  fresh and powdered, for recipes, 20
  Garlic-Herb Roasted Beef Tenderloin, 66
  Garlic-Peppercorn Cream Sauce, 93
  Garlic-Rosemary Compound Butter, 127
  Garlic-Rosemary Filet Mignon, 30–31
  London Broil, 87–88
  Mongolian Beef, 58–59
  Red Curry Steak and Vegetable Kebabs, 70–71
  Slow Cooker Garlic-Herb Filet Mignon and Potatoes, 69
  Smoked Paprika and Garlic Aioli, 118
Gas grills, 28

Ginger
  Ginger-Soy Sirloin Steak Roll-Ups, 74–75
  Mongolian Beef, 58–59
  Red Curry Steak and Vegetable Kebabs, 70–71
Grain-fed beef, 16
Grass-fed beef, 16
Gravy, White Country, 125
Grilled Flank Steak with Corn-Avocado Salsa, 76–77
Grilled Lamb Chops with Spicy Sesame-Peanut Sauce, 108
Grilled Tofu Steak with Chimichurri Sauce, 98
Grilled Tri-Tip with Chimichurri Sauce, 80
Grilling
  indoors (stovetop), 32
  outdoors, 28–29
Grills
  charcoal, 28, 29
  gas, 28
  outdoor, 19
Ground beef. *See also* Plant-based ground beef
  Salisbury Steak with Mushroom Gravy, 107

H

Ham
  Brown Sugar and Maple-Dijon Ham Steak, 103
  Honey Mustard Ham Steak Panini with Havarti Cheese, 104
Hanger steak
  about, 10

Chile-Lime Hanger Steak Tacos, 90
Sweet and Spicy Grilled Hanger Steak, 92
Herbs. *See also specific herbs*
Chimichurri Sauce, 122
Hollandaise Sauce, Smoky, 124
Homestyle Mashed Potatoes, 114
Honey Mustard Ham Steak Panini with Havarti Cheese, 104
Horseradish Garlic Sauce, Creamy, 119

I

IPA-Marinated Grilled Pork Steak with Sweet and Tangy Steak Sauce, 102

K

Kebabs, Red Curry Steak and Vegetable, 70–71
Kitchen tools, 18–19
Knives, 18, 19
Kobe beef, 16

L

Lamb Chops, Grilled, with Spicy Sesame-Peanut Sauce, 108
Lemon-Pepper Compound Butter, 33
Lettuce
  Black and Blue Grilled Steak Salad, 55
  Romaine Salad with Garlic and White Wine Vinaigrette, 117
London Broil, 87–88

M

Maillard reaction, 35
Maple-Dijon and Brown Sugar Ham Steak, 103
Marinated Flank Steak, 83
Marinating steaks, 21
Mongolian Beef, 58–59
Montreal Grilled Rib Eye with Sautéed Balsamic Mushrooms and Onions, 68
Mushrooms
  Classic Beef Stroganoff, 91
  Creamy Peppercorn-Mushroom Sauce, 126
  Creamy Steak Alfredo Pasta, 61
  Montreal Grilled Rib Eye with Sautéed Balsamic Mushrooms and Onions, 68
  Peppercorn-Mushroom Sauce, 52–53
  Salisbury Steak with Mushroom Gravy, 107
  Sautéed Balsamic Mushrooms and Onions, 115
  Sous Vide Rib Eye Steaks with Sautéed Mushrooms and Balsamic Vinegar Sauce, 62–63
  Steak Diane, 64
  Swiss Steak, 89
Mustard
  Brown Sugar and Maple-Dijon Ham Steak, 103
  Honey Mustard Ham Steak Panini with Havarti Cheese, 104

N

Natural beef, defined, 16
Noodles, Ramen, Steak and Broccoli with, 81

O

Olive oil, 20
Onions
   Montreal Grilled Rib Eye with Sautéed Balsamic Mushrooms and Onions, 68
   Philly Cheesesteak Sandwiches, 56–57
   Pressure Cooker Skirt Steak Fajitas, 95
   Red Curry Steak and Vegetable Kebabs, 70–71
   Sautéed Balsamic Mushrooms and Onions, 115
Organic beef, defined, 16
Oven-Baked Steak Fries, 112
Oven mitts, 18
Oven-Roasted Prime Rib with Horseradish Sauce, 65

P

Panini, Honey Mustard Ham Steak, with Havarti Cheese, 104
Pan-Seared Filet Mignon, 37
Pan-Seared New York Strip with Garlic-Rosemary Compound Butter, 50
Pan-searing steak, 34
Paprika, Smoked, and Garlic Aioli, 118
Parchment paper, 18
Paring knife, 19
Pasta, Creamy Steak Alfredo, 61
Peanut-Sesame Sauce, Spicy, Grilled Lamb Chops with, 108
Pepper
   Creamy Peppercorn-Mushroom Sauce, 126
   Garlic-Peppercorn Cream Sauce, 93
   Lemon-Pepper Compound Butter, 33
   Peppercorn-Mushroom Sauce, 52–53
   types of, 20
Peppers (bell). *See also* Chile peppers
   Flat Iron Steak Stir-Fry with Asparagus and Red Pepper, 84–85
   Pressure Cooker Skirt Steak Fajitas, 95
   Red Curry Steak and Vegetable Kebabs, 70–71
   Slow Cooker Pepper Steak, 82
Philly Cheesesteak Sandwiches, 56–57
Plant-based ground beef
   Sous Vide Vegan Steak, 99
Plastic bags, 19
Pork. *See also* Bacon
   Brown Sugar and Maple-Dijon Ham Steak, 103
   Honey Mustard Ham Steak Panini with Havarti Cheese, 104
   IPA-Marinated Grilled Pork Steak with Sweet and Tangy Steak Sauce, 102
Porterhouse steak
   about, 7
   Porterhouse Steak with Creamy Peppercorn-Mushroom Sauce, 52–53
Potatoes
   Homestyle Mashed Potatoes, 114
   Oven-Baked Steak Fries, 112
   Slow Cooker Garlic-Herb Filet Mignon and Potatoes, 69
   Twice-Baked Potatoes, 113
Pressure cooker, 19
Pressure Cooker Skirt Steak Fajitas, 95
Prime grade, 17
Prime rib
   Oven-Roasted Prime Rib with Horseradish Sauce, 65

Slow Cooker French Dip
    Sandwiches au Jus, 67

R

Ramen Noodles, Steak and Broccoli
    with, 81
Red Curry Steak and Vegetable
    Kebabs, 70–71
Reverse searing steak, 35
Rib eye steak
  about, 6
  Creamy Steak Alfredo Pasta, 61
  Deep-Fried Boneless Rib Eye, 43
  Mongolian Beef, 58–59
  Montreal Grilled Rib Eye with Sautéed
    Balsamic Mushrooms and Onions, 68
  Philly Cheesesteak Sandwiches, 56–57
  Sous Vide Rib Eye Steaks with
    Sautéed Mushrooms and
    Balsamic Vinegar Sauce, 62–63
  Southwestern Steak Stew, 60
Romaine Salad with Garlic and White
    Wine Vinaigrette, 117
Rosemary
  fresh and dried, 20
  Garlic-Rosemary Compound Butter, 127
  Garlic-Rosemary Filet Mignon, 30–31
  London Broil, 87–88
Round steak
  Slow Cooker Pepper Steak, 82

S

Salads
  Black and Blue Grilled Steak Salad, 55
  Brussels Sprout Salad with Bacon and
    Balsamic-Dijon Vinaigrette, 116
  Romaine Salad with Garlic and
    White Wine Vinaigrette, 117
Salisbury Steak with Mushroom
    Gravy, 107
Salmon Steak Fillet with Citrus-Cucumber
    Salsa, 100
Salsa
  Citrus-Cucumber Salsa, 100
  Corn-Avocado Salsa, 76
Salt, 20
Sandwiches
  Honey Mustard Ham Steak Panini
    with Havarti Cheese, 104
  Philly Cheesesteak Sandwiches, 56–57
  Slow Cooker French Dip
    Sandwiches au Jus, 67
Sauces
  Béarnaise Sauce, 120–121
  Chimichurri Sauce, 122
  Creamy Garlic Horseradish Sauce, 119
  Creamy Peppercorn-
    Mushroom Sauce, 126
  Garlic-Peppercorn Cream Sauce, 93
  Peppercorn-Mushroom Sauce, 52–53
  Smoked Paprika and Garlic Aioli, 118
  Smoky Hollandaise Sauce, 124
  Sweet and Tangy Steak Sauce, 123
  White Country Gravy, 125
Sautéed Balsamic Mushrooms and
    Onions, 115
Sautéing steak, 35
Scoring steaks, 21
Seasoning steaks, 21
Select grade, 17
Sesame-Peanut Sauce, Spicy, Grilled Lamb
    Chops with, 108

Sirloin steak
  about, 8
  Classic Beef Stroganoff, 91
  Ginger-Soy Sirloin Steak
    Roll-Ups, 74–75
  Lemon-Pepper Petite Sirloin, 33
Skillet, cast-iron, 18
Skirt steak
  about, 10
  Pressure Cooker Skirt Steak Fajitas, 95
  Spicy Southwest Cocoa-
    Rubbed Skirt Steak, 86
  Steak and Broccoli with
    Ramen Noodles, 81
Slow Cooker French Dip Sandwiches
  au Jus, 67
Slow Cooker Garlic-Herb Filet Mignon
  and Potatoes, 69
Slow Cooker Pepper Steak, 82
Smoked Paprika and Garlic Aioli, 118
Smoked Tri-Tip, 94
Smokers, 19, 29
Smoky Hollandaise Sauce, 124
Sous vide method, 40
Sous Vide New York Strip Steak, 41
Sous vide precision cooker and
  container, 19
Sous Vide Rib Eye Steaks with Sautéed
  Mushrooms and Balsamic Vinegar
  Sauce, 62–63
Sous Vide Vegan Steak, 99
Southwestern Steak Stew, 60
Spicy Southwest Cocoa-Rubbed Skirt
  Steak, 86
Steak (beef). *See also specific steak cuts*
  beef grades, 17
  broiling, 36
  butcher's steaks, about, 4
  butcher's steaks, list of recipes, 73
  checking internal temperature, 22–23
  cooked, reheating, 24
  cooked, storing, 23
  cooking sous vide, 40
  cutting against the grain, 20
  deep-frying, 42
  defined, 4
  doneness chart, 22
  filet mignon, about, 7
  flank, about, 9
  flat iron, about, 9
  hanger, about, 10
  kitchen tools for, 18–19
  knife skills for, 20–21
  outdoor grilling, 28–29
  pan-searing, 34
  pantry ingredients for, 20
  premium, list of recipes, 49
  premium cuts, about, 4
  raw, storing, 23
  reverse searing, 35
  rib eye, about, 6
  sautéing, 35
  seasoning and marinating, 21
  sensory cues, 17
  shopping for, 17–18
  sirloin, about, 8
  skirt, about, 10
  stovetop grilling, 32
  T-bone/porterhouse, about, 7
  terms used with, 16
  trimming fat from, 21
  tri-tip, about, 8

Steak (other)
   Ahi Tuna with Lemon-Pepper Compound Butter, 101
   Brown Sugar and Maple-Dijon Ham Steak, 103
   Grilled Lamb Chops with Spicy Sesame-Peanut Sauce, 108
   Grilled Tofu Steak with Chimichurri Sauce, 98
   Honey Mustard Ham Steak Panini with Havarti Cheese, 104
   IPA-Marinated Grilled Pork Steak with Sweet and Tangy Steak Sauce, 102
   Salmon Steak Fillet with Citrus-Cucumber Salsa, 100
   Sous Vide Vegan Steak, 99
Steak Sauce, Sweet and Tangy, 123
Steak tartare
   about, 44
   recipe for, 45
Stew, Southwestern Steak, 60
Strip steak
   Black and Blue Grilled Steak Salad, 55
   Creamy Cajun Steak Bites, 54
   Pan-Seared New York Strip with Garlic-Rosemary Compound Butter, 50
   Red Curry Steak and Vegetable Kebabs, 70–71
   Sous Vide New York Strip Steak, 41
Stroganoff, Classic Beef, 91
Sweet and Spicy Grilled Hanger Steak, 92
Sweet and Tangy Steak Sauce, 123
Swiss Steak, 89

T

Tacos, Chile-Lime Hanger Steak, 90
T-bone steak
   about, 7
   T-Bone Steak with Béarnaise Sauce, 51
Tenderloin, Beef, Garlic-Herb Roasted, 66
Thermometer, 18
Thyme, 20
Tofu Steak, Grilled, with Chimichurri Sauce, 98
Tomatoes
   Black and Blue Grilled Steak Salad, 55
   Southwestern Steak Stew, 60
   Swiss Steak, 89
Tongs, 19
Tri-tip steak
   about, 8
   Grilled Tri-Tip with Chimichurri Sauce, 80
   Smoked Tri-Tip, 94
Twice-Baked Potatoes, 113

U

USDA Prime, Choice, and Select, 17

V

Vacuum sealer, 19
Vegan Steak, Sous Vide, 99

W

Wagyu beef, 16
White Country Gravy, 125

Z

Zucchini
   Ginger-Soy Sirloin Steak Roll-Ups, 74–75

Acknowledgments

To God be the glory! A special thanks to my husband, Greg Mason, who supports me always. I'm lucky to have you. To my daughter, Kyliegh Mason, who gave me the support and help I needed to finish this book. To my son, Davis Mason, who encouraged me while I wrote and cooked. Kyliegh and Davis, thank you for being taste testers, providing valuable feedback, and being a huge support. I leave you a legacy. I love you all forever.

To my mom, Kathy Peach, who taught me to be a strong woman, to always go big—and just go. I am forever thankful—that mind-set changed my life and opened uncountable doors. To my dad, Bobby Peach, who tasted just about every recipe for this book. Thank you for your feedback, loyalty, and support. I am forever grateful. To my nephew, Tyree Hardge, one of my biggest supporters, who pushes me to go bigger. I dedicate this book to you. I love you all.

To my best friend Jennifer Stem, one of my biggest cheerleaders for more than 20 years. You, Bo, and the kiddos are family. I would not be who I am today without your love and support. I love you. I'm forever grateful.

To my best friend Holly Wilson, who supports me even though we are 3,000 miles apart—for 20+ years. I love you. You are family. I'm forever grateful.

To my dear friend Lyndsay Pineda, who supports me from across the pond. Your encouragement and words have affected me like no one has. I'm forever thankful!

To Anthony Vargas and Lisa Miles (Mama Lisa), you are family, and no matter what, I love you. Your support and faithfulness mean everything. I am forever thankful.

To the brother I never had, Tyler Bain, your efforts, engagements, and support with *Recipes Worth Repeating* and Amanda Mason Photography speak volumes. I am so thankful! We love you!

To Bill and Heather Huberich, thank you for supporting me and being amazing taste testers. You are our family; we love you!

Jami, Dallas, Gage, and Daisha Berger, thank you for being test tasters. I love your sweet family!

To Eddie, Rita, Adam, and Kiana Wong, thank you for always being ready, willing, and available to test recipes! Your feedback ensures so many people will enjoy these recipes even more because of you!

To Neal, Amy, Rees, Gia, and Kingston Jones, thank you for sticking by my side as I created these recipes, for your feedback, your kitchen, and your time. You are our family. We love you.

To Lexie Miller and Jackson Moore (Let's GO!), thank you for being taste testers and giving me feedback!

To John Blakely (Blake) and Chris Franz, without your trust in me and support in all I do, I could not have accomplished this. You have changed my family's life—thank you.

To my amazing editor, Anna. Thank you and the editorial staff for making this book possible.

To my readers and supporters at *Recipes Worth Repeating*, this book is possible because of you. I am forever thankful!

About the Author

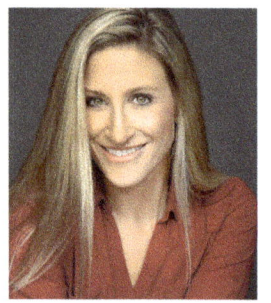

AMANDA MASON is the author of *Smoking Meat Made Easy* and the founder and creator of *Recipes Worth Repeating*, a food blog featuring family-focused recipes since 2012. Amanda began cooking at a young age. After she started working at a local restaurant, Franklin Chop House, as a teenager, her passion for cooking and food preparation grew. Her recipes and writings have been featured in *Taste of Home* and on MSN, SheKnows.com, BravoTV.com, and many more print and online outlets. Born and raised near Nashville, Tennessee, she now lives with her husband and two children in Phoenix, Arizona. Visit her website: RecipesWorthRepeating.com.

www.ingramcontent.com/pod-product-compliance
Lightning Source LLC
LaVergne TN
LVHW070948070426
835507LV00029B/3457